Suicide and Self-Injury in Schools

Interventions for School Mental Health Specialists

DARCY HAAG GRANELLO
PAUL F. GRANELLO
GERALD A. JUHNKE

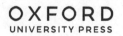

OXFORD
UNIVERSITY PRESS

OXFORD
UNIVERSITY PRESS

Oxford University Press is a department of the University of Oxford. It furthers the University's objective of excellence in research, scholarship, and education by publishing worldwide. Oxford is a registered trade mark of Oxford University Press in the UK and certain other countries.

Published in the United States of America by Oxford University Press 198 Madison Avenue, New York, NY 10016, United States of America.

© Oxford University Press 2023

All rights reserved. No part of this publication may be reproduced, stored in a retrieval system, or transmitted, in any form or by any means, without the prior permission in writing of Oxford University Press, or as expressly permitted by law, by license, or under terms agreed with the appropriate reproduction rights organization. Inquiries concerning reproduction outside the scope of the above should be sent to the Rights Department, Oxford University Press, at the address above.

You must not circulate this work in any other form and you must impose this same condition on any acquirer.

Library of Congress Cataloging-in-Publication Data
Names: Granello, Darcy Haag, author. | Granello, Paul F., author. | Juhnke, Gerald A., author.
Title: Suicide and self-injury in schools : interventions for school mental health specialists / Darcy Haag Granello, Paul F. Granello, Gerald A. Juhnke.
Description: New York, NY : Oxford University Press, [2023] | Includes index.
Identifiers: LCCN 2022030905 (print) | LCCN 2022030906 (ebook) | ISBN 9780190059842 (paperback) | ISBN 9780190059866 (epub)
Subjects: LCSH: Students—Suicidal behavior. | Teenagers—Suicidal behavior. | Suicide—Prevention. | Adolescent psychology. | School psychology.
Classification: LCC HV6545.8 .G73 2022 (print) | LCC HV6545.8 (ebook) | DDC 362.280835—dc23/eng/20220801
LC record available at https://lccn.loc.gov/2022030905
LC ebook record available at https://lccn.loc.gov/2022030906

DOI: 10.1093/oso/9780190059842.001.0001

Disclaimer: The resources in this book are intended for use only as a tool to assist clinicians/school-based professionals and should not be used to replace clinical judgment or school-based policies and procedures. The information in this book is not provided as legal advice and/or professional advice on specific situations. While we have attempted to ensure the accuracy of information contained herein, we do not warrant that it is complete or accurate, and we are not legally responsible for errors or omissions.

1 3 5 7 9 8 6 4 2

Printed by Marquis, Canada

Suicide and Self-Injury in Schools

Contents

The Premise of This Book: A Comprehensive Strategy for Suicide Prevention

Welcome! It is an honor to have you review the opening pages of our book, *Suicide and Self-Injury in Schools*. With the turmoil of the last few years—the pandemic and the social, political, economic, and racial upheaval—more students than ever are coming to school in psychological distress, and more students than ever are at risk for suicide. School mental health professionals must step up to meet this demand, at a time when they themselves are already overburdened and perhaps struggling with their own mental health as they too face the demands the last few years have placed on us all.

The foundational principle of this book, however, is that with proper planning and a core team to assist, you won't have to face this on your own. In fact, we argue that *you can't and in fact shouldn't do this alone*. This book will give you the strategies for how to create a team, develop a plan, and, together, develop a Comprehensive School-Based Suicide Prevention Program. This book is a how-to guide, with over 120 practical, hands-on strategies to get you started.

Chapters 2 and 3 of the book will help you gain a better understanding of who in your school might be at highest risk. As these high-risk groups of students are identified, specific, practical, and evidence-based strategies are introduced that can be used to help address suicide risk in culturally, developmentally, and individually appropriate ways. In Chapter 4, we turn our attention to the effects of social media and the role that technology plays in understanding suicide risk among students. This chapter includes over a dozen specific strategies that schools can adopt right now (and some strategies for parents too!). In Chapter 5, we take on the important topic of self-injury and its complicated relationship to suicide. Because of the large numbers of students who engage in self-injury in schools, this chapter includes 16 practical strategies for working with these students. Beginning with Chapter 6, and throughout the remainder of the book, we discuss how to plan and implement a comprehensive suicide prevention program, including a model with 10 components that include all three tiers of prevention programming. In each of these chapters, each time we introduce a critical component of the plan, we will give you evidence-based strategies with hands-on approaches, often providing specific words, websites, models, and methods to use.

We know the entire process can feel overwhelming. Our job is to help make this feel more manageable, more doable, and more in your control—to help you envision yourself leading a team that will develop and implement this plan. We all know it is important, and we believe that a conceptual map, with lots of clear strategies to help you fill in each step, will help you get to where you want to be.

Of course, you have other resources to help guide you too. As a school-based mental health professional or administrator, you have your professional associations to offer assistance. The American School Counselor Association (ASCA), National Association of School Psychologists (NASP), National Association of School Nurses (NASN), School Social Worker Association of America (SSWAA), and National Association of School Secondary Principals (NASSP) all have resources and guidelines that can help you as you work to keep your students safe.

Finally, we want to remind you that you are the expert on your students, families, and community. Although we offer a lot of research-based concepts and practices, we hope that you use these ideas appropriately for your school. Integrate what makes sense. We don't want to eclipse your own expertise or clinical knowledge.

It is not our intent to tell you what to do or what will work with your students. The book is designed to offer guidance as you respond to the unique needs of your students. The pages you read are potential strategies designed to empower your students, your schools, your families, your community, and you.

We sincerely thank you for allowing us the privilege of serving you as you respond to the crisis we are all facing—the escalating suicide risk of our students. We truly wish you the very best in your professional efforts to protect and help America's students and tomorrow's leaders.

Darcy Haag Granello
Paul F. Granello
Gerald "Jerry" A. Juhnke

Warning

Addressing suicide risk and self-injury is a complex process. It is literally impossible to identify all students who might be suicidal. Thus, any assessments or face-to-face interviews described in this book should not be used as the sole method to make a suicide risk assessment or intervention. There are no suicide risk assessments that have been empirically validated to assess risk with any certainty. Students who are suicidal should be continually re-evaluated by an experienced interdisciplinary mental health team. Parents/guardians should always be notified if a student is suicidal, regardless of level of risk. Comprehensive suicide risk assessments should be completed by mental health professionals (typically off-site) who are specifically trained to complete these assessments. Remember: Always consult your mental health supervisor, school district legal counsel, professional liability insurance risk management carrier, professional peers, and assigned school police or safety officers to ensure the greatest degree of safety and ultimate protection. Consult school policy regarding decisions for return to school after hospital stays. Any decisions related to this population should never be made by one individual.

Acknowledgments

We have spent the last 25 years walking the path of suicide prevention. Some days are filled with unbearable pain and heartbreak, and some days are filled with stories of hope and perseverance. But there is one thing that every day has in common: We have shared every day on this journey with others who are on the same path. For 25 years, we have found kindred spirits who wake up every day knowing that they will spend the day doing everything in their power to help prevent suicide. It is for you that we have written this book. We are so grateful to have you share this journey with us. To each of you—the counselors, school psychologists, nurses, social workers, principals, teachers, and all of the staff who reach out, every day, to the students who are hurting and to the families and loved ones of those we have lost—we are grateful for the work that you do and for the people you are. To the parents, students, bus drivers, custodians, and lunch ladies—you make a difference. You notice. You care. We are grateful to have you with us on this journey too. You remind each student that they matter. They are worth it. They deserve to be happy. To the students who are in pain and are suffering—we hope you hold on. Our sincere intent is that this book helps someone in your life get this message to you: There is help. There is hope.

We also extend our gratitude to those who fill our lives with joys and blessings, to those who care for us, who bring us laughter and cheer, and who remind us that even in the darkest of times, there are always brighter days ahead. Thank you to our friends and colleagues who lift our spirits when we need it the most, including

Brian and Kristin Haag, Tracee and Roddy Meade, Erica and Jeff Carter, Jo Gehringer, Jenn and Robb Pentico, and D. J. Todd.

We would also like to thank Ms. Laura Lewis of the Ohio State University Suicide Prevention Program for her expertise and the kindness with which she shares it. To Mr. Dana Bliss and the Oxford University Press team, we thank you all for your publication support and skill.

Finally, we want to thank our families, who stand with us in good times and sorrow and help us stay grounded and feel loved as we continue to engage in this important work. Thank you, Alanna, Kevin, Brian, Victor, Matt, Debbie, Bryce, and Brenna.

1

A Call to Action

Children and adolescents are at risk for suicidal thoughts and behaviors. They lack adult perspective and experience, and many have not yet learned to handle life's challenges. Today, children and adolescents face situations or exposure to information or images that are developmentally beyond their capacity to understand or manage. Coupled with life during a time of increasing political and racial divisiveness, economic struggles, and the challenges of growing up during a pandemic, it is not hard to understand why our young people are struggling.

It is not just young people, however, who cannot keep pace with these changes. In our fast-moving world, our adult understanding of child and adolescent suicide is desperately trying to keep up with the daily onslaught of new information and advice that can feel overwhelming, or even contradictory. It can make even those of us who want to help feel uncertain about what is the "best" or "right" thing to do. You may find yourself among those who are searching for some clear and practical guidelines to help you get started—and that is perhaps why you find yourself reading these words. The good news is that giving you some concrete steps is precisely what this book is designed to do. The even better news is that if you are reading this book, chances are that you, like many others, now recognize that there is no time to waste.

Yet it wasn't always so. Up until the last decade or so, there was a rather universal belief among many adults that made it easy to minimize suicide risk in young people. There was a rather persistent myth that for *most* children, childhood is a carefree time with little worry or responsibility. Adults compared the stressors that

Suicide and Self-Injury in Schools. Darcy Haag Granello, Paul F. Granello, Gerald A. Juhnke,
Oxford University Press. © Oxford University Press 2023. DOI: 10.1093/oso/9780190059842.003.0001

children faced to the challenges that they faced in their own adult lives, or they remembered their own childhood through proverbial rose-colored glasses. As we traveled the country talking about suicide risk in children and adolescents, we heard time and again that although this was certainly a possibility among *some* children and teenagers, for *most* young people this was a reality far from imaginable. When we spoke with school administrators about the national rates of students who had suicidal thoughts or attempts in an effort to try to encourage suicide prevention programming at the local level, we heard time and time again, "Not in my school" or "We have good kids."

In recent years, however, we have found in our conversations with parents and school professionals that the opposite beliefs have begun to take hold. Suddenly, there has been a dramatic shift. Many adults now believe that childhood and adolescence are so fraught with dangers and drama that suicide, mental health disorders, addictions, and trauma seem nearly inevitable. When the pandemic struck in 2020, the situation became even more bleak. Whereas we once had to struggle to convince people to hear the message that our children are at risk, we now find that it can be a struggle to convince people that there is something that can be done to help. We now must convince them that we can help foster resilience and hope in a generation of young people facing new challenges—and new opportunities. Adults, still using their same adult perspectives, view the world of social media, technology, and the entire information age and see how it overwhelms and engulfs our children. Living through the changes in the educational system and the increased mental health needs of children and adolescents that came with the pandemic and quarantine caused even higher levels of concern. Parents, school personnel, and even the children and adolescents themselves struggle to make sense of the new reality without becoming discouraged and hopeless.

The truth, of course, lies somewhere in the middle. Just as it always has been, childhood and adolescence are both a time of joy and possibilities and a tumultuous period that can elicit thoughts, emotions, and experiences that are extremely difficult to manage. Children and adolescents often have little control over their situations at home, at school, and increasingly online. They may not have the coping skills, knowledge, or opportunities to seek help when they need it the most. When young people do want help, they often don't know where to turn. Ironically, in a world that offers the lure of unlimited knowledge and information, navigating the resources can create a new form of paralysis.

We begin this book with a discussion of some of the most common problems and concerns related to child and adolescent suicide. In the coming chapters, we will share some of the most frequently occurring stressors and try to understand the role these problems play that contribute to suicide or other self-injurious behaviors. Although the tone of this book in general will be more about proactive and positive approaches to suicide prevention and intervention, we believe it is important to start here. Most professionals (and many parents) believe they have an overall sense of the problem, but in our experience, every person—every professional, every parent, every graduate student, every administrator, every mental health professional, every member of the media, every politician, in short, *everyone*—we encounter has been stunned and shocked by some of this information. The effect of all of this information, compiled together, can be disturbing and alarming and can have a jarring effect on readers. We caution you before you start that this can be difficult to read. The good news is, the rest of the book will give you some practical action plans to put into place. But first, take a deep breath as you dive into some of the darker realities that today's children and adolescents face.

A Look at the Numbers: Putting It Into Perspective

In 2020 suicide was the 12th leading cause of death for all ages in the United States. However, for people between the ages of 10 and

24, suicide was the third leading cause of death, accounting for over 6,000 deaths in this age bracket each year (Drapeau & McIntosh, 2021). That is equivalent to more than 16 suicides per day, or one suicide every 90 minutes. Although suicide deaths represent just 1.4% of all deaths in the United States. each year, suicide accounts for 17% of all deaths among 15–24-year-olds. That is because young people are far less likely to die than older adults. But when young people do die, it is far more likely to be by their own hand. Think about this for a moment. Among young people, *nearly one in five who dies does so by suicide.*

The 10–24 age group represents a wide developmental continuum, and as might be expected, there are large variations in rates of suicide attempts and completions, as well as methods within this group. In general, within this age group, as people mature, they are more likely to die by suicide. This means that traditional college-age students (20–24 age group) are nearly twice as likely to die by suicide as high school students. It also means that high school students (15–19 age group) are 6 times more likely than middle schoolers (10–14 age group) to die by suicide. It is worth noting, however, that these numbers are starting to change. More and more, younger and younger students are dying by their own hand. Between 2006 and 2017, according to the Centers for Disease Control and Prevention (CDC), the suicide rate among middle and high schoolers *increased by 70%* (Hedegaard et al., 2018). We will come back to this in a few moments and we will repeat it again, because in our experience, it is worth repeating, and statistics like these need time to truly sink in.

Between 2006 and 2017, the suicide rate for youth age 10–17 increased by 70%.

And, of course, that statistic was *before* the pandemic and quarantine.

Suicide Ideation and Suicide Attempts

Suicide deaths, however, represent only one extreme end of the continuum of suicidal thoughts and behaviors. More people think about, talk about, plan for, and attempt suicide during adolescence than during any other life stage, and they desperately need our help. In the 10–24 age group, there are more suicide attempts for every suicide completion than in any other age group. We are just now beginning to fully understand the sheer magnitude of these numbers. Although estimates of attempts have varied widely over the years, it is widely believed that there are as many as 200–300 suicide attempts per suicide death among young people. One study found that there are an estimated *5,240 suicide attempts each day* by young people in grades 7–12, or *nearly 2 million suicide attempts each year* (Jason Foundation, 2017). Many of these attempts have low lethality and do not require medical attention. Nevertheless, every year, approximately 970,000 youth between the ages of 5 and 17 receive medical care for their suicide attempts at emergency departments across the United States (Burstein et al., 2019). It is worth noting that this number has *more than doubled* since 2007.

National surveys of high school students (grades 9–12) in public and private schools consistently find high levels of suicide ideation and behaviors. The CDC uses its National Youth Risk Behavior Surveillance System (YRBSS) to survey more than 14,000 students in 144 schools each year to better understand a multitude of health risk behaviors among America's students. In 2019, the results of the YRBSS (CDC, 2019) found that within the past year, among high school students:

- 18.8% seriously considered suicide,
- 15.7% created a suicide plan,
- 8.9% reported trying to take their own life, and
- 2.5% reported a suicide attempt that was severe enough to require medical attention

This represents a significant increase over the last decade.

The YRBSS surveys of middle school students in 2017 (CDC, 2017; grades (6–8) in public and private schools consistently show similarly disturbing numbers:

- Seriously thought about killing themselves
  - 16.2% of sixth graders
  - 19.5% of seventh graders
  - 22.9% of eighth graders
- Made a suicide plan
  - 9% of sixth graders
  - 12.8% of seventh graders
  - 16% of eighth graders
- Made a suicide attempt
  - 6.6% of sixth graders
  - 7.6% of seventh graders
  - 9.3% of eighth graders

It is important to note that not all states participate in the Middle School Youth Risk Behavior Surveillance, and the rates reported vary widely from state to state among those states that do participate in this survey. Nevertheless, *overall* trends are clear. The suicide rate among middle school students *doubled* between 2007 and 2014, and the rates of ideation, plans, and attempts are also increasing at an alarming rate among this age group. In 2014, for the first time in U.S. history, the death rate from suicide surpassed that from car crashes in the 10–14 age group (CDC, 2016).

We encourage you to take a moment to stop and put these statistics into your own frame of reference. How many students are there in the school where you work, where you are an intern, or where your child is a student? We often think about this in terms of a "typical" high school with 1,000 students. In that high school, in the last year, 188 students seriously thought about suicide, 157 developed a plan, 89 had an attempt, and nearly 25 were taken to the hospital or required other medical assistance. Clearly, suicide, suicide ideation, and suicidal behaviors represent a very real and very significant public health problem among the nation's young people.

We are only a few pages into this book, and for many readers, you may have already found a statistic that surprised or alarmed you.

- Nearly one in five deaths among young people is a suicide.
- Between 2006 and 2017, the death rate by suicide for youth age 10–17 increased by 70%.
- There are over 5,000 suicide attempts *a day* in grades 7–12.
- Nearly 19% of high school students seriously consider suicide.

What do you want to remember?

Making Sense of the Statistics

As troubling as all these statistics are, they are probably low. Many suicides are ruled as accidental deaths. Often, accidents are often associated with recklessness and/or alcohol use, which are also suicide risk factors. Drug overdoses, for example, are often recorded as accidental deaths but could actually be unrecognized suicides. There are countless stories of single car crashes, falls from buildings, poisonings, and even gun violence that require coroners to make a final determination of death. Without clear evidence that the death was intentional, and when faced with grieving families, there is often pressure to rule deaths as accidents. In spite of a public perception that suicide notes are common (fostered, perhaps, by movies and the media), as few as 15% of people who die by suicide leave a note (Callanan & Davis, 2009). Without a note and without clear suicidal intent, coroners often classify the death as accidental. Researchers agree that suicide in the United States is underreported by as much as 50%, with even higher rates of misclassification among youth suicide (Shepard et al., 2015). Using this metric, it may well be that we lose closer to 14,000 young American lives to suicide each year.

In our work with training school personnel and other professionals about suicide, we have found that the data and statistics can quickly become overwhelming, leaving us all with a sense of despair and hopelessness. You may be feeling that sense of dismay as well. The sad truth is that suicide rates among young people are increasing, and exposure to suicide ideation and attempts in school has become nearly routine for far too many schoolteachers, administrators, counselors, school psychologists, and staff. Perhaps, then, it should come as no surprise that when we are exposed to these figures, our natural tendency is to feel helpless. The frustration and fear that we all have around the topic of child and adolescent suicide clearly aligns with some of the concerns we all have about larger social problems that face today's youth. And although the information can be overwhelming, it is important to take some time and reflect on the implications this has for all of us as individuals—whether we are mental health professionals, administrators, educators, or family members and friends. Each of us can do something to help prevent suicide. If we become educated and informed and are willing to educate others, intervene when needed, and seek help when appropriate, we can help make a difference.

Practical strategy (self-awareness): Recognize your own reactions to the topic of adolescent suicide. Common reactions include fear, anxiety, anger, and helplessness. Note that these emotional reactions can lead to unproductive and unhelpful choices, such as deciding not to talk about suicide at the individual or school level, denying the level of suicide risk of the students in your school, or deciding to leave all discussions, planning, and programs about suicide to someone else, often to an individual school counselor, but sometimes to a school principal or to an outside resource that comes into a school and engages in a one-shot suicide prevention program.

The Pandemic and Teen Suicide

It will be several years before we have a full understanding of the effects the pandemic and quarantine have had on child and adolescent suicide and mental health. Nevertheless, it is clear that there were sharp increases in anxiety and depression among all segments of the U.S. population that occurred shortly after the COVID lockdowns began in March of 2020. School-aged children and adolescents were particularly hard hit. They were cut off from their peers and many of the caring adults in their lives (such as their teachers, coaches, and counselors), unable to experience many of the normal "rites of passage" (such as prom and graduation), faced with uncertain futures, and in homes where many had access to lethal weapons, and school mental health professionals began to express concern that suicide rates among this group would rise. By June of 2020, approximately one in four American teenagers had suicidal thoughts. Hotlines began to see spikes in calls from middle- and high-school-age students, and mental health professionals saw significant increases in depression and anxiety in this age group. When schools began to reopen, teachers and school mental health professionals started to see students who were exhausted, scared, hopeless, and anxious. In addition, they found that the staff in the building, who were facing the same uncertainty and challenges, had difficulty meeting the increased demand for help. A spring 2021 survey of over 200,000 students at 585 schools in 19 states found that in the spring of 2020 (prepandemic), 39% of students said that feeling depressed, anxious, or stressed was an obstacle to learning. Just 1 year later, that number had increased to 49%. During that same time period, 46% of students said that they believed there was an adult in the school that they could talk to when they were feeling stressed or having problems. Again, just 1 year later, postpandemic, that number decreased to 39% (YouthTruthSurvey.org, 2021). In other words, as more and more students were feeling overwhelmed, depressed, and anxious, fewer students believed that there was an adult at the school that they could reach out to about their problems. Clearly, we have a problem.

What is less clear are the long-lasting effects that living through the pandemic and the disruption it caused will have on this generation of young people. As schools scrambled to adapt to the immediate needs of their students, administrators and mental health professionals began thinking about the long-term implications. We are thinking about that too.

What Is *Your* Role in This?

We often hear people say that they are not "expert enough" to participate in suicide prevention in schools. No matter how much training or experience anyone has on the topic, we know that it can feel overwhelming. It is easy to think someone else in the building should be in charge or is better prepared, and suicide prevention is best left to others. Unfortunately, that approach doesn't work. Everyone has to learn. Everyone has a role to play. We fundamentally believe (and have research to demonstrate) that suicide prevention works best when we take a team approach. This is *not* something that can be left only to the school counselor or the crisis intervention team. Yes, there may be a mental health professional in the building or district who leads the way, but when it comes to suicide prevention, it is *essential* that every staff member work together—from the principal and administrative staff to the teachers, classroom aides, custodians, and people who serve the lunches. Creating a culture of care in a school building or district can save lives and means that **Suicide Prevention Is a Shared Responsibility**.

Throughout the remaining chapters of this book, we will give you the tools to provide everyone in the district and in the building (and that includes parents) the concrete action steps they need to feel part of this important work.

A Quick Primer in Language

Before we move on, it's important to find a common language for all of the different aspects of suicidal thoughts and behaviors. The words we use matter. Words influence people's attitudes, and attitudes determine behaviors. Within the world of suicide prevention, it is critical that we use the words that communicate effectively exactly what we mean to say to others about a specific student or situation. It is also important that we do so in a way that increases the likelihood that each individual student feels heard, respected, and valued.

Use Person-First Language

First and foremost, we advocate for person-first language. This means that we never use a person's mental illness or suicidal state as a noun. We never define a person as equivalent to a label (e.g., "he is mentally ill" or "she is bipolar"). Not only is this dehumanizing and reductionistic, but also research clearly demonstrates that within the field of mental health, using labels such as these to describe individuals (e.g., schizophrenic vs. person with schizophrenia) results in much lower levels of tolerance, perceived worth, and willingness to ascribe even basic levels of humanity to the other individual (see Garcia et al., 2020; Granello; 2019; Granello & Gibbs, 2016; Granello & Gorby, 2021). Although it may be tempting to use these linguistic shortcuts among professionals with the implicit understanding that "we know what we mean," we can never do this. It may surprise you to learn that of all the different groups measured in these studies (undergraduates, members of the general population, practicing counselors, counseling students), mental health professionals were the *most* affected by the choice of language. That is, when we take this shorthand approach to labeling our students and clients as their diagnoses, rather than using person-first language, we begin to treat them as *less than* the people they are.

Use the Term "Suicide Death" or "Suicide"

When describing a death, try to avoid ascribing motives or making assumptions. We will discuss ways to report on or discuss suicide in Chapter 10 when we discuss suicide postvention, including ways to discuss suicide deaths with the media. For now, it is important to know that for the purposes of this book, when we discuss suicide, we mean self-directed self-injurious behavior with the intent to die as a result of that behavior.

Don't Say "Committed Suicide." It's a common term, we know, but one that carries a strong moral overtone. After all, the word "commit" is usually used with some other sort of moral choice (think "commit adultery," "commit a felony," or "commit a sin"). It probably is not surprising, then, that there is a strong pushback within the community of individuals who have had their lives impacted by suicide to resist this term.

While we're at it, here are some other words to avoid:

Don't Say "Successful Suicide." Of course, there is nothing successful about a suicide, or for that matter, nothing unsuccessful or failed about an attempt that didn't lead to a death.

Don't Say "Suicidal Gesture" or "Manipulative." Simply describe the behavior. "Suicidal gesture" is an outdated term that was often used to minimize an individual's talk of suicide or their suicide attempts. Words like "gesture" or "manipulate" make it easy for us to ignore people's actions instead of taking them seriously. "Parasuicide" is another term that is generally considered outdated. It was once used to describe a nonlethal suicide attempt. We know it is tempting to interpret some of the behaviors that some individuals display in this way, but it certainly does not lead to quality care. We will talk more about this in Chapters 8 and 9, but for now it is important to remember that the way we discuss the behaviors in which people engage *greatly affects* the way they are treated.

Other Suicide-Related Terminology

Like every field, the world of suicidology has its own language, which is evolving and by no means universally agreed upon (if you are really interested in some of these detailed discussions, here are some starting places: Brenner et al., 2011; Silverman et al., 2007). For most of us, the level of detail in these discussions may be interesting (or not, depending on your fascination with both suicide and lexicography), but it is probably unnecessary. Here are some of the terms that you will need to know as you use this book.

Suicide Attempt.   A suicide attempt is a nonfatal, self-directed, potentially injurious behavior with the intent to die as a result of the behavior. A suicide attempt may or may not result in injury, and an injury may or may not be severe. The crucial aspect of a suicide attempt is *the person's intent to die.* It is the individual belief that the attempt will be lethal (regardless of the actual lethality of the attempt) that results in the classification of a behavior as a suicide attempt. We have had this argument with emergency room physicians who have refused to classify a child or adolescent's behavior as a suicide attempt because the young person simply did not select a lethal medication or consume the medication in sufficient quantity, even though there was a clear intent to die. For example, a person might ingest a half bottle full of antidepressants, thinking it will kill them, and they are rushed to the hospital, only to learn that an overdose on this medication will typically not lead to death. Failure to classify such cases as suicide attempts only means that the person will not receive the appropriate intervention and that the next time they are suicidal, a simple Internet search will give them the information they need to ensure that they consume a sufficiently lethal dose of the "right" medication.

Suicidal Behaviors. Because there are many other types of suicidal behaviors that can lead up to an attempt that has the intent of lethality, the term "suicidal behaviors" is used as a catch-all to encompass a lot of different acts. Essentially, suicidal behaviors include anything beyond verbalizations or thoughts, including preparing for suicide (sometimes called preparatory acts, such as buying a gun, collecting pills, writing a suicide note, or giving away prized possessions). The American Psychiatric Association includes the term "aborted suicide attempt" in this category. This includes behaviors such as climbing to the top of a building or holding a gun to one's head but not following through with the attempt.

Suicidal Thoughts/Suicide Ideation. These words refer to thinking about, considering, or planning suicide. This is a broad category that contains all of the thoughts that people have about suicide. This can range from passive thoughts about wanting to be dead to active thoughts about killing oneself but stop short of any behaviors, such as developing a suicide plan.

Suicide Plan. The development of a suicide plan involves a proposed method for carrying out a plan of action that will ultimately lead to one's death.

Suicide Loss Survivor/Survivor of Suicide Loss. In general, these are the terms used to define anyone who has lost a loved one to suicide. The term "suicide survivor" is less clear. It is sometimes used by people who have lost a loved one to suicide, and it is sometimes used by individuals who have survived a suicide attempt, although those individuals may describe themselves as "suicide attempt survivors." Because the term "suicide survivor" is ambiguous, we recommend that you use either "suicide loss survivor" or "suicide attempt survivor," and these are the terms that we will use in this book.

Nonsuicidal Self-Injury (NSSI). NSSI (or often just self-injury) is the act of deliberately engaging in self-harm. NSSI often involves acts such as cutting, burning, or punching oneself, although there are many different ways that people may engage in self-harm. The link between NSSI and suicide is unclear, and this may be because there are many different reasons people engage in NSSI behaviors. For many people, NSSI is a way to manage severe emotional pain, anger, loneliness, or frustration. Although NSSI is intended to bring calm and release tension, it is often followed by intense shame and guilt and a return of the emotion. Rates for NSSI vary greatly by age, gender, sexual orientation, and a number of psychosocial stressors, such as bullying victimization, substance use, and depression. *In general*, females and students who are LGBTQI+ individuals engage in NSSI at higher rates, and high school students engage in NSSI more often than middle-school- or elementary-aged students. Because there is a clear but complicated link between NSSI and suicide, we will discuss NSSI throughout this book, and we have devoted an entire chapter to NSSI (see Chapter 5).

Moving Forward

Normally, chapters end with conclusions. In this case, however, this is just the beginning, and it is time to get started. Perhaps with no other age group do we find ourselves so in need of action. Although young people do not have the highest rates of suicide, their deaths strike us as particularly painful. Their deaths represent a loss of potential that is hard to accept. In fact, one of the ways that suicide is represented in government statistics is through something called "years of potential life lost (YPLL)." When young people die by suicide, it's hard not to think of all of their potential that we have lost, of all that the future could have held, and of all the possibilities that will never come to fruition. When we lose young people, we lose all the contributions they could have made. Perhaps they would have grown up to become scientists or inventors who would have solved society's problems, politicians or diplomats who would have promoted peace and understanding, or loving fathers, mothers, brothers, sisters, and partners who would have changed the face of a family. Whatever their future, we lose their potential and their possibilities, making these deaths particularly hard to bear. There's no time to waste. Let's get started.

References

Brenner, L. A., Breshears, R. E., Betthauser, L. M., Bellon, K. K., Holman, E., Harwood, J. E., Silverman, M. M., Huggins, J., & Nagamoto, H. T. (2011). Implementation of a suicide nomenclature within two VA healthcare settings. *Journal of Clinical Psychology in Medical Settings, 18*(2), 116–128. doi:10.1007/s10880-011-9240-9

Burstein, B., Agostino, H., & Greenfield, B. (2019). Suicidal attempts and ideation among children and adolescents in U.S. emergency departments, 2007–2015. *JAMA Pediatrics, 173*(6), 598–600. doi:10.1001/jamapediatrics.2019.0464

Callanan, V. J., & Davis, M. S. (2009). A comparison of suicide note writers with suicides who did not leave notes. *Suicide and Life-Threatening Behavior, 39*(5), 558–568.

Centers for Disease Control and Prevention. (2016). QuickStats: Death rates for motor vehicle traffic injury, suicide, and homicide among children and adolescents aged 10–14 years—United States, 1999–2014. *MMWR Morbidity and Mortality Weekly Report, 65,* 1203. http://dx.doi.org/10.15585/mmwr.mm6543a8

Centers for Disease Control and Prevention. (2017). *Middle school youth risk behavior surveillance—United States, 2017.* U.S. Department of Health and Human Services.

Centers for Disease Control and Prevention. (2019). *Suicide ideation and behaviors among high school students—Youth Risk Behavior Survey—United States, 2019.* U.S. Department of Health and Human Services.

Drapeau, C. W., & McIntosh, J. L. (2021, December 24). *U.S.A. suicide: 2020 Official final data.* Suicide Awareness Voices of Education (SAVE). https://save.org/wp-content/uploads/2022/01/2020datapgsv1a.pdf

Garcia, G., Granello, D. H., & Boehm, K. (2020). At last: Empirical proof that the "R-word" really must go: The influence of terminology on tolerance. *Inclusion, 8*(2), 155–162. doi:10.1352/2326-6988-8.2.155

Granello, D. H. (2019). The "R-word" is more than hate speech: Differences in counselors' level of tolerance based on language and labels. *Journal of Humanistic Counseling, 58,* 170–183.

Granello, D. H., & Gibbs, T. A. (2016). The power of language and labels: "The mentally ill" versus "person with mental illness." *Journal of Counseling and Development, 94*, 31–40.

Granello, D. H., & Gorby, S. R. (2021). It's time for counselors to modify our language: It matters when we call our clients schizophrenics vs. people with schizophrenia. *Journal of Counseling and Development, 99*, 452–461.

Hedegaard, H., Curtin, S. C., & Warner, M. (2018). Suicide rates in the United States continue to increase. *NCHS Data Brief, no. 309*. National Center for Health Statistics.

Jason Foundation. (2017). *Youth suicide statistics.* https://jasonfoundation.com/youth-suicide/facts-stats/

Shepard, D. S., Gurewich, D., Lwin, A. K., Reed, G. A., & Silverman, M. M. (2015). Suicide and suicidal attempts in the United States: Costs and policy implications. *Suicide and Life Threatening Behavior, 46*(3), 352–362.

Silverman, M. M., Berman, A. L., Sanddal, N. D., O'Carroll, P. W., & Joiner, T. E. (2007). Rebuilding the Tower of Babel: A revised nomenclature for the study of suicide and suicidal behaviors. *Suicide and Life-Threatening Behaviors, 37*(3), 264–277.

YouthTruthSurvey.org. (2021). *Students weigh in: Part III: Learning and wellbeing during COVID-19.* https://youthtruthsurvey.org

2

Understanding Who Is at Risk

After even the most cursory glance at the first chapter, it should be clear to you that suicide is a significant—and growing—problem in schools across the country. However, there are differences in risk among students based on the demographic group to which they belong. In this chapter, we will discuss who is at risk, based on their membership in these groups. Understanding some of the basics of these risk categories can help school mental health specialists, administrators, and staff recognize students who, by virtue of their inclusion in a particular demographic category, might be at elevated risk—and provide programming and support to help students in these groups navigate these challenges.

We believe that it is important to include this information and for school personnel involved in suicide prevention to have a basic understanding of how sex, gender, race, and age affect risk. However, we also know that we must be extremely careful. Demographic information is useful, but it is important to remember that no demographic group is a monolith. There are *wide variations* within each group. More importantly, students who belong to a certain demographic group "on paper" may, in fact, identify with that group very little, if at all, in practice. Nevertheless, we offer the following broad brushstrokes about some major demographic categories and their suicide risk.

Sex and Gender

Sex describes the biological sex a person was assigned at birth. Gender is a social construct that is based either on the social role

Suicide and Self-Injury in Schools. Darcy Haag Granello, Paul F. Granello, Gerald A. Juhnke, Oxford University Press. © Oxford University Press 2023. DOI: 10.1093/oso/9780190059842.003.0002

assigned by others based on sex (gender role) or on the person's own identification of gender (gender identity). In suicide prevention research and programming with children and adolescents, the terms "sex" and "gender" have often been used interchangeably, which can make it difficult to understand the lived experiences of transgender children and gender-fluid students. In this book, we will be careful to use the words male/female when we mean biological sex and boy/girl or man/woman when we mean gender. When possible and available, we will also make note of when research differentiates between sex and gender.

There is a well-known sex and gender paradox in suicide. Girls and women (as well as females) do everything related to suicide more than men, boys, and males, with only one notable exception. Women and girls think about, talk about, and attempt suicide more than men and boys. But when it comes to suicide death, men and boys are far more likely to die by their own hand. This has been true historically and remains true across every nearly every country on earth where suicide is documented, with only China recording suicide rates for men and women in near-equal ratios. In every other country in the world, including the United States, the sex and gender paradox remains remarkably consistent across all age groups, all races, and all social classes.

Boys Are at Higher Risk of Dying

Historically, boys and men have been nearly 4 times more likely to die from suicide than girls and women. This boy/man-to-girl/woman ratio has been remarkably consistent across all age groups in the U.S. population for decades. Across all age groups in 2020, more than 79% of all suicide deaths were by boys/men (Drapeau & McIntosh, 2021). However, in the last decade, we have begun to see the beginnings of a change. More and more girls, particularly in middle school, are dying by suicide. The historic sex/gender gap in suicide deaths, at least for these young students, has been closing. Among the 10–14-year-old age group, the boy-to-girl suicide death ratio is far lower, closer to 2:1 (Centers for Disease Control and Prevention [CDC], 2018b). It is important to note that suicide deaths among middle-school-aged children are still relatively rare, and care should be taken not to extrapolate too far into the future with these numbers. In other words, just because the gap is closing for middle school children does not mean that by the time these children reach adulthood, the ratio between the sexes will remain at this historic low. Nevertheless, it is clearly an important trend that deserves attention.

In spite of this recent uptick in suicide deaths among middle school girls, it is clear that overall, men and boys are at higher risk for suicide death. This probably does not come as a surprise to you, and there have been many hypotheses that have been put forward about the higher rates of suicide death by boys and men. As you think about your own reactions to this information, you undoubtedly can come up with your own reasons about why boys and men might be at higher risk. In the paragraphs that follow, we have listed some of the most common reasons for this gender gap in suicide, but this list, of course, is by no means exhaustive.

Boys Choose More Lethal Means. Certainly lethality is one reason that men are more likely to die by suicide. In general, boys and men tend to choose more lethal means, such as firearms, whereas girls and women are more likely to choose pills or poisons. Nearly 40% of U.S. children live in a home with at least one gun, and more than a third of those homes have an unlocked gun (J. Kim, 2018). Simply put, firearms allow less time for intervention. Given the high rates of impulsivity that often accompany the suicides of young men and boys in particular, firearms carry a particular threat. At least one take-home message is that locking up guns and ammunition is a necessary, but not sufficient, strategy to reduce adolescent suicide. One of the more chilling comments we have heard was from a young man when he told us,

"The only thing that stopped me that day was that I couldn't find the bullets."

Practical strategy (parents): It is not uncommon for families with guns in the home to be resistant to giving up those guns, even if a child is at high risk for suicide. We have found that asking a family to remove guns from the home is rarely successful. A more useful strategy might be to encourage the family to give the guns to a trusted friend or family member, for a specified period of time, during the suicidal crisis. We have found that families are far more likely to comply. We might say to a parent, for example:

"Would you be willing to give the guns to your brother (or another trusted adult) to lock up in his home during this crisis? This is only temporary while [child] is in suicidal crisis. When the crisis is over, probably in 4–6 weeks [or whatever timeline is deemed appropriate], then the guns can be returned to your home, properly and safely stored, of course."

Boys Are Socialized Not to Seek Help. In this explanation, biological sex and gender role socialization clearly overlap. Across all ages, men and boys have fewer social support systems, and those who are socialized as male are less likely to seek mental health care. The gender disparity in help seeking has been well documented. In general, the more men and boys internalize traditional gender role expectations, the less likely they are to seek psychological help (e.g., Juvrud & Rennels, 2017; Wahto & Swift, 2016).

The traditional gendered socialization of men and boys encourages risk-taking behaviors, self-sufficiency, independence, and emotional control. There is ample evidence that adolescent boys, more than girls, engage in cigarette smoking, including the use of e-cigarettes; binge drinking; drug use (all types); fighting; antisocial behavior; aggression; and violence (e.g., CDC, 2019; Reyes et al., 2016). Each of these behaviors is an independent risk factor for suicide. Taken together, it is hardly surprising that boys are at higher risk for suicide. Additionally, boys are socialized to be less comfortable reporting and seeking help for their problems, and they may be more inclined to believe that it is more adult, more "manly," to handle problems on their own.

More and more, we are hearing from young people (and adults too) that developing a healthy sense of masculinity may be more difficult today than it has been in the past. As far back as 1985, Brannon outlined core themes that run through the lives of traditional males that make it more difficult for them to seek counseling when needed. In 1985, Brannon argued that these themes were already so entrenched in the culture that it was incredibly challenging for any individual male to fight them. The four themes are as follows:

1. *No Sissy Stuff.* Boys are often raised to believe that they must be masculine. Any signs of emotional vulnerability or help seeking are labeled as feminine and, therefore, devalued and avoided.
2. *The Big Wheel.* In this traditional upbringing, boys are raised to believe that masculinity is equated with power, ambition, and success. Once boys become adults, this is also called the "breadwinner bind," whereby men are socialized to believe they must work as hard as possible to provide the best life for their families and then are criticized for neglecting family responsibilities because of their work commitments.
3. *The Sturdy Oak.* Boys raised to follow this definition of masculinity value rational and logical thought over emotions. They may not have been taught to recognize or acknowledge emotions, or may even have been taught to deny or fear them.
4. *Give 'Em Hell!* This theme of masculinity emphasizes the need to seek adventure, excitement, and risk, even through the use of violence. Boys raised to glorify this type of masculinity value not only physical strength and toughness but also aggression and "winning at all costs."

Although there are clearly changes in the way boys are being raised since Brannon wrote about these four themes more than three decades ago, the essence of these themes is still part of male socialization. What is perhaps more challenging for our current generation of young men is that they are raised in a culture that has not yet completely shed these old expectations and simultaneously not yet developed new expectations for behavior. The phrase "toxic masculinity" is now used to define these old stereotypes, yet there are no new clear models for them to follow. Think about all the different messages that you hear on a daily basis about what it means to be a man. Is it one of the action superheroes in the latest blockbuster movie? A sports figure? A social media celebrity? A bachelor in a rose ceremony? Maybe it isn't too surprising that our boys are having a hard time finding role models to help them navigate the transition to manhood.

In fact, in a 2014 survey, when presented with a very long list of options, more than 40% of the male respondents could not find anyone on the list they could identify as a potential role model. Of those who did select a male role model, just under a third (30%) selected their father, and grandfather came in second (at 7%). At least to some extent, this suggests that males often have difficulty identifying male role models. Although this study was done in the United Kingdom, there is little reason to believe that the results would be significantly different in the United States (Welford & Powell, 2014).

Practical strategy (schools): Because male students are less likely to engage in help-seeking behaviors, it may be particularly important to develop school-based strategies to encourage male students to seek help. Vocal and visible male role models within the school (male teachers, coaches, counselors, parents, older students) who openly discuss and normalize mental health concerns and encourage help-seeking behaviors may be particularly important. Some studies have highlighted the importance of encouraging boys in particular to be active participants in suicide prevention efforts. Therefore, it might be even more effective if boys in the school were to help identify the men in the school who could be role models that would be most influential within the school system, which could help make this cultural shift.

Boys' Brains Are Not Yet Fully Developed.   A third explanation for higher risk of death among adolescent boys concerns neurodevelopmental issues that most certainly play a role. The development of the adolescent brain (particularly the prefrontal and limbic circuitry) influences risk-taking and impulsivity, both of which are associated with suicide risk. Adolescent brain development differs by biological sex (Auerbach et al., 2017), and it may be that boys' brains are simply wired to be more impulsive and less developmentally prepared to handle the complexity of modern adolescent life.

Girls Are at Higher Risk for Suicidal Ideation and Attempts

Although boys die by suicide more often, girls tell us that they think about suicide, plan for suicide, and attempt suicide at rates that are at least 2–3 times higher than boys (CDC, 2019). However, it is becoming increasingly clear that suicide deaths by young girls are on the rise. Teenage girls account for a small portion of all the suicide deaths each year, but the suicide rate for young girls (age 10–14) is the fastest growing in the nation, tripling from 2000 to 2015. It is unclear what is behind this trend.

As you think about the rise in suicide deaths and the high rates of suicidal thoughts, plans, and attempts in young girls, you may have your own ideas about what is contributing to this trend. In the following paragraphs, we list some ideas that may contribute to this phenomenon, but there are no definitive answers. As always, we encourage you to continue to be vigilant as you keep up with strategies to address this growing problem.

Girls Have Higher Rates of Depression. There are high rates of depression among young girls. Over 41% of high school girls report that they have had persistent feelings of hopeless and depression during the last year, and rates of depression among young girls have tripled by 59% over the last decade (CDC, 2017). Some have blamed the high rates of depression on the earlier onset of puberty, as the increase in and fluctuating levels of hormones associated with the menstrual cycle can contribute to and exacerbate depressive symptoms (Bichell, 2016). Others have presented different reasons for the rise in depression in girls, such as the pressure to fit in, to get good grades, and the effects of technology. Finally, although we do not yet fully understand how the pandemic has affected the long-term mental health of the children who lived through it, initial results of multiple studies all conclude the pandemic was particularly hard on girls (Racine et al., 2021). Across the globe, girls had higher rates of depression during the pandemic, often double what they were prior to the pandemic. The effects of social isolation, missed milestones, school disruptions, family financial and social struggles, and the loss of structural and personal support from school are all possible reasons for the devastating effects on girls.

In spite of the rapid increase in the numbers of young girls who meet criteria for major depression, there is a rather widespread reluctance among many parents and even some health professionals to take depression seriously in young girls. Perhaps because so many young girls say they feel this way, it can begin to feel like it is the new normal, or just an expected part of puberty. It may be that the failure to distinguish clinical depression from normal adolescent moodiness is at least part of the reason that 62% of adolescents with depression *never receive any treatment* (Mental Health America, 2018). Left untreated, a depressive episode can last an entire academic year.

Practical strategy (schools): Helping students, parents, and teachers recognize the difference between normal adolescent moodiness and the symptoms of clinical depression can help those in need receive treatment. Simple education that highlights key differences such as duration (moodiness seldom lasts longer than 2 weeks without any noticeable breaks, yet 2 weeks is required for a diagnosis of depression), severity (clinical depression is more severe and has a greater effect on functioning), and domain (clinical depression is typically not domain specific but occurs in multiple areas of the child's life, such as home and school, and in interactions with friends and family) can help. There are other important educational aspects to understanding clinical depression that would be helpful for students, parents, and teachers to understand.

Girls Spend More Time on Social Media.   In several large-scale studies that have drawn a lot of media attention, girls' suicide risk has been correlated to time spent on social media. Teenage girls who spend more time on social media each day are more likely to have at least one suicide-related outcome, such as depression, thinking about suicide, developing a suicide plan, or having an attempt. Nearly half of teenage girls who indicated they spent 5 or more hours a day on a smartphone, laptop, or tablet said they had contemplated, planned, or attempted suicide at least once—compared with 28% of those who said they spend less than an hour a day on a device. These same studies found that there appears to be a cutoff point at about 2 hours a day, with teenagers who spend less than 2 hours a day on social media not having the same level of negative outcomes. Additionally, although boys are also affected by social media, they do not, in general, tend to spend as much time on social media, instead spending their time on games or other Internet activities that do not appear to have the same effects (Twenge et al., 2018). Because social media is such an important aspect of suicide prevention in the current environment, we dedicate an entire chapter to this topic (see Chapter 4).

Practical strategy (parents): We understand that limiting social media to 2 hours per day may be difficult, but this is supported by research. Further, insisting that phones be left outside the bedroom to encourage a better night's sleep can help reduce the negative effects of social media on depression and suicide. We recognize that this is a daunting task. Nevertheless, the implications of unrestricted time spent on social media, particularly for young girls, cannot be ignored. Researchers also recommend having clear discussions with adolescents not only about how much time they can spend on social media but also about what they are allowed to do once they are on there (e.g., Twenge et al., 2018).

Transgender Youth Are at Highest Risk

Transgender youth have much higher rates of all suicide thoughts and attempts than their cisgender peers (those whose gender identity aligns with their sex assigned at birth). As many as 50% of transgender adolescents report a suicide attempt at some point during their lives (Toomy et al., 2018). The highest rates of attempts are among transgender, female-to-male adolescents and among gender nonbinary youth, although rates among all transgender populations are significantly elevated. During the pandemic, more than 83% of gender nonbinary youth stated that they felt so depressed, stressed, or anxious that they had difficultly learning in school, making them the students with the highest level of distress (YouthTruthSurvey.org, 2021). Of course, suicidality and depression among trans youth is incredibly complex, involving social, systemic, and structural oppression.

Strategies to improve the mental health and well-being of trans youth can have a significant impact on reducing suicidal thoughts, attempts, and deaths in this age group. Of course, as school systems work to promote the mental health of their trans youth, they must operate within the legal requirements of their state and with the awareness of the specific social climate and context of their schools. For example, as of early 2022, 64 bills had been introduced around the United States that were specifically designed to deny gender-affirming medical treatments to trans youth. According to the Trevor Project, the simple fact that these bills (and the 400+ other anti-LGBTQI+ bills introduced in 2021) are being debated by state legislatures, regardless of outcome, has significantly and negatively affected the mental health of trans youth. For example, the Trevor Project reported that crisis contacts from LGBTQ youth increased 150% from 2020 to 2021, with many transgender and nonbinary youth stating they were "feeling stressed, using self-harm, and considering suicide due to anti-LGBTQ laws being debated in their state" (Gruberg & Medina, 2022). We know this is complicated, and there are no easy answers. Nevertheless, recognizing the significant need for mental health assistance for these students is an important first step.

Unfortunately, trans youth are often grouped with students who are lesbian, gay, and bisexual (e.g., the term "LGBT"), which confuses sexual orientation with gender identity. The result can be that the needs of trans youth, who are often in the numerical minority in a school, can be overlooked.

Practical strategy (schools): Much of the work to help improve the mental health of trans students will require efforts to fight systemic oppression. Some strategies, however, are small and relatively easy to implement but have large impacts. Allowing trans youth to choose the name by which they are called in school has been associated with a 29% decrease in suicidal thoughts, as well as an associated decrease in depression and in suicidal behavior (Russell et al., 2018).

Sexual Orientation

Just as with trans youth, there is ample evidence that across the entire lifespan, people who identify as lesbian, gay, bisexual, queer, questioning, or other orientations (LGBQQ+) live in environments that are typically immensely and chronically distressing and op-pressive, with discrimination that takes the form of personal re-jection, hostility, harassment, bullying, and physical violence. Additionally, minority stress theory posits that individuals of marginalized identities (including LGBQQ+ youth) experience chronic stress, internalized bias (in the form of internalized ho-mophobia), and societal pressure to uphold oppressive norms (Hatchel et al., 2019). Among LGB youth who are rejected by their parents or other family members, suicide risk is even higher. LGB youth from highly rejecting families are 8 times more likely to at-tempt suicide (CDC, 2016). All major health and mental health pro-fessional associations have taken a stand against any therapies or interventions designed to change the sexual orientation or gender identity of anyone under the age of 18, which is sometimes called "conversion therapy," although there is pushback against this term, as it is argued that it legitimizes this practice as a type of therapy when, in fact, there is no empirical evidence to support its use. Many states (20 states as of early 2022) are adopting laws to ban the practice of change efforts (conversion therapy) by any licensed professionals.

Lesbian, Gay, and Bisexual Youth Have Higher Ideation, Attempts, and Deaths

Suicide is the *leading cause of death* among children and adolescents who identify as LGB. Although it is difficult to obtain information about the sexual orientation of young people who die by suicide, it may be that as many as one in four teenagers who dies by suicide identifies as LGB (Ream, 2019), and LGB youth attempt suicide more than 4 times as often as non-LGB students (CDC, 2019). The elevated risk for suicidal thoughts and suicidal behaviors among LGB youth has been a consistent pattern among all research studies for middle and high school students and, in more recent research, in elementary students as young as age 9 (Blashill & Calzo, 2019).

It is particularly important for mental health professionals, administrators, and teachers in middle and high schools to recognize the suicide risk for LGB students because, although risk is elevated throughout life, it appears that the greatest risk is during times of coming out. For most (although certainly not all) LGB people, this occurs during the teenage and young adult years. The risk is higher still if the youth is outed involuntarily (Haas et al., 2010). We are not surprised that this is a time of elevated risk. Coming out is associated with increased rates of depression, isolation, bullying, and substance use, all of which are independent risk factors for suicide. Having said that, it is also important to say that for most people, "coming out" is not a singular moment or an event, but a process that is complex and occurs multiple times with different people or groups.

In our conversations with LGB youth, we are careful to be very clear that there is *nothing inherent about a person's sexual orientation that increases suicide risk*. We have found that all too often, LGB youth are well aware of the statistics about suicide, and they might believe that their orientation condemns them to a lifetime of suicidal thoughts and behaviors, depression, and pain. It is *exceedingly important* that messages given to LGB youth (and to everyone in the school) emphasize that it is the societal context surrounding these youth (as well as trans, nonbinary, and questioning students) that elevates the risk, and that there is nothing intrinsic to being LGB that increases suicide risk. From our experience, if we don't take time to help make this distinction, our discussion of suicide risk with LGB students can inadvertently contribute to the internalized homophobia that these students already may feel. In addition, we have found that helping LGB students recognize that although there will always be people in their lives who may be homophobic or unaccepting, they will not always be in middle or high school. It is for this reason that campaigns such as "It Gets Better" have been so powerful, with more than 50,000 videos on the website and more than 50 million views. Although campaigns such as these have been criticized for being overly simplistic, it is also clear that giving these students hope for the future while simultaneously creating a school climate that promotes and celebrates all students, and has zero tolerance for bullying, is an appropriate multipronged effort to reducing suicide thoughts and behaviors among students who identify as LGBQQ+.

Practical strategy (schools): A positive school climate has been associated with decreased depression, suicidal feelings, substance use, and unexcused school absences among LGBQI+ students. Importantly, LGB students who say they feel connected to at least one adult (any adult in the school) have lower rates of suicidal behaviors. For LGB students, having an adult in the school to talk to serves as a protective factor against suicide attempts, even for students who are bullied at school or online. In other words, LGB youth who experienced bullying (cyber or in person) had much higher rates of suicide attempts unless they had an identified adult at the school they could talk to (Duong & Bradshaw, 2014).

Clearly, making sure that LGB students have a specific and identified individual adult source of support is essential. It is our experience from talking with students that it is not sufficient to say, "You can talk to the school counselor" (and research will back this up). Rather, each student must identify the individual adult who is that student's support person (remember, it might be a teacher; a staff person, including a custodian, bus driver, or lunch server; or a member of the administrative staff). The critical piece is that this is the student's decision. We believe it is important to facilitate initial conversations between the student and the support person and set some initial guidelines. For example, a typical protocol is that the student and the support person agree to at least make brief contact with each other every day and have a quick conversation. This is important because it enhances connectedness. It also means that when the student needs to have a difficult conversation or needs help, they not only have an identified person in the school but also do not have to figure out how to break the ice and start a conversation.

Practical strategy (schools): The idea that one doesn't have any real meaningful relationships or belong to any real groups (called "thwarted belongingness" in the interpersonal theory of suicide) is particularly important for teenagers who identify as LGBTQI+ . Thwarted belongingness is characterized by loneliness and isolation, and it has been linked to higher levels of suicidal behaviors in LGBTQI+ students. There is evidence that in schools with LGB support groups (such as GSAs, or gay-straight alliances), LGB students are less likely to experience threats of violence, miss school because they feel unsafe, or have suicide thoughts or attempts than those students in schools without LGB support groups (Goodenow et al., 2006; Saewcy et al., 2014). Importantly, LGB students in schools with GSAs report higher perceived levels of social support, although more recent studies have made it clear that GSAs work best when they are housed in schools with overall positive and accepting climates and when participating students are motivated and engaged (Calzo et al., 2020). Nevertheless, student groups that promote positive interactions between LGB and non-LGB students and contribute to an overall positive climate within the school are believed to help prevent suicidal behaviors because students are more likely to talk to peers than to adults if they are contemplating suicide. In this way, these groups help buffer against feelings of thwarted belongingness, thereby serving as an important protective factor against suicide for LGB students (Hatzenbuehler et al., 2014).

Practical strategy (parents): How parents respond to their LGBTQI+ teen can have a tremendous impact on their adolescent's current and future mental well-being and suicide risk. Schools can help parents link to local, state, and national organizations and resources to learn how they can help support their LGBTQ+ student.

Race

Suicide affects members of all races, although there are differences in suicide deaths and attempts based on race. Among young people, just as with all age groups, some of these racial differences intersect with other group characteristics, most notably sex. Thus, it is difficult to make blanket statements about the effects of race on suicide for young people. For example, American Indian/Alaska Native (AI/AN) boys have the highest rates of suicide death, and Black/African American girls have the lowest rates (although this is starting to change). By sheer numbers, Caucasian/White boys are the most likely to die by suicide.

Practical strategy (schools): It is important for mental health professionals within each school to have an understanding of the specific risk for their students. It is clearly beyond the scope of this book (or any book) to include the suicide risk factors for every demographic group. For example, two of the authors (Darcy and Paul) live in a community with a large Somali population. Before any school-based suicide prevention programming can occur, it is essential to understand the risk factors that are most relevant for the students in the building. Of course, one of the best ways to do this is through the local community resources, including the community mental health, neighborhood, and religious associations, who understand the suicide risk factors that need to be addressed within the school and are sensitive to the cultural norms.

American Indian/Alaska Native Populations Are at the Highest Risk, With Boys Having the Highest Rates

Suicide rates for AI/AN adolescent populations are twice as high as for their same-aged non-Native peers. The gender paradox that holds true for the adolescent population in general is also apparent among AI/AN students.

Despair Is a Significant Risk Factor. It appears that AI/AN young people are no more likely than others their same age to think about suicide, but they are *far more likely* to engage in suicidal behaviors (Qiao & Bell, 2017). It is unclear why this is true, although the most common reasons that have been suggested are the modeling of suicidal behaviors by adults in the community, lack of access and opportunities for education, higher rates of alcohol use, greater access to firearms, and lack of access to effective mental health care. What also appears to be the case is that AI/AN adolescents are more likely to engage in cluster suicides, or to have suicide contagion. That is, because these adolescents tend to live in more closed communities (either on reservations or to be more isolated from their peers within schools, spending more time in the company of each other), they are more affected by the suicide death by one of their AI/AN peers.

> Practical strategy (schools): Mental health professionals must recognize that AI/AN students seem to be more susceptible than others to impulsive suicides (e.g., more likely to have an attempt if they think about suicide). The implications are that there needs to be high support during critical moments (e.g., access to suicide hotlines) and strong efforts for means restriction (e.g., locking up guns and pills). Further, because of the heightened risk for contagion among AI/AN students, postvention programming and mental health surveillance of all AI/AN students following the death of a fellow student are essential.

Asians/Pacific Islanders Are at Elevated Risk and Are, in General, Less Likely to Seek Help

It is difficult to say much with any certainty about suicide risk among the Asian American adolescent community, primarily because we use the term "Asian American" to represent people from many different countries with many different perspectives about suicide. In fact, according to the U.S. Census Bureau, there are 43 different ethnic subgroups with about 100 different languages and dialects that are represented under the umbrella term "Asian American" (CDC, 2017). This makes it difficult to make sweeping generalizations about Asian Americans and suicide.

In spite of these challenges, it is clear that Asian American youth are, in general, at elevated risk for suicide death. About a third of all deaths among the 15–24 age group are by suicide, making suicide the leading cause of death for Asian American youth, the only demographic group for whom this is true (CDC, 2018). Across the diversity of the youth that fit into the label "Asian American," there are several key risk factors that consistently rise to the surface.

Family Relationships Play a Significant Role. Asian American youth, in general, tend to have higher levels of depression when they have very different levels of acculturation than their parents. When children perceive that their parents are clinging to the "old ways" or holding them to standards from the "old country" and children are not embracing these same customs, this increases the tension and conflict in the home. This is true whether or not the parents are first-generation immigrants. Nevertheless, most experts agree that Asian American youth have higher levels of positive mental health outcomes when they retain at least some aspects of their heritage or ethnic identity, including, but not limited to, minimal language competency (Choi et al., 2018). It may be that when children retain at least some remnants of their ancestral culture, there is less of a perceived gap between the generations.

Young Asian American students also may perceive that their parents engage in a different parenting style than that which they see displayed in Western media or in the homes of their non–Asian American friends. For example, they may perceive that their parents are less emotional or more distant. In general, Asian American youth who believe that their parents are supportive and emotionally present are less likely to exhibit symptoms of depression and more likely to remain psychologically well adjusted over time.

In addition, some (although certainly not all) Asian American children face high academic expectations, a push to succeed at all costs, and parental expectations for narrow or predetermined career or academic pathways. This can increase the level of parent-child conflict and contribute to adolescent depression. The much-publicized (and much-criticized) term "tiger parenting" has come to be synonymous with this type of parenting. For these parents, there is a belief that academic achievement comes from hard work more than from innate cognitive ability, and this leads to more and more time devoted to schoolwork.

Clearly, navigating cultural expectations, such as obligations to parents and families, while finding a balance between collectivist and individualist values can be a significant challenge for many Asian American youth. Learning to bridge this cultural gap has no easy answer, and for many young people, the result is an increased risk for depression and suicide.

Practical strategy (schools): Any strategy that schools use to help Asian American students must first and foremost recognize and respect the diversity within this population, recognizing that a single approach cannot possibly meet the needs of students from more than 50 different countries of origin, 20 different major religions, and a large range of sociocultural experiences. One strategy that may be helpful, in conjunction with others, is to help Asian American students navigate an identity that plays on the strengths of both their Asian and American identities. This may be particularly important for students who are first-generation or who have parents who are first-generation immigrants. Rather than selecting either culture, helping students and their parents work together (with community resources, as appropriate) to take the best from both cultures can be an important step in learning how to talk about mental health and suicide and can open the conversation in a way that both participants can honor and understand.

Difficulties in Peer Relationships Can Greatly Exacerbate Risk. Of course, childhood and adolescence can be a difficult time for many young people as they learn to navigate peer relationships. However, for many Asian American youth, there are several challenges that may make peer relationships even more difficult to manage.

For first-generation Asian American students, orientation to the U.S. culture can be particularly difficult, made even more challenging by the necessity of learning English. Asian American students with low English proficiency are far more likely to be discriminated against or bullied by their peers (S. Y. Kim et al., 2011). Family stressors, such as parental pressure to focus on academics, may mean that for some Asian American students, there is less time available for peer socialization or engagement in other school extracurricular activities. This can lead to isolation or racial segregation, both of which have been associated with higher rates of bullying and depression.

Black/African American Youth Are at Increasing Risk, Particularly Among the Youngest Children

In general, Black youth have lower rates of suicide death than the national average for their same-age peers, and Black girls have the lowest rates of suicide deaths. However, there have been some drastic changes in recent years that point to some disturbing trends. Suicide rates for all Black youth have been on rise, but the greatest increase in rates has been among the very young.

Get Started Early. Elementary-age Black children (ages 5–11) now die at rates that are more than double the national average (Price & Khubchandani, 2019). Among urban Black children, there is at least some evidence that the highest risk for suicide ideation is during middle school, regardless of gender (seventh grade; Musci, 2016). Taken together, this information makes it clear that suicide prevention programming for Black children must start early in their academic careers.

Practical strategy (schools): Children who die by suicide are more likely than adolescents to have a diagnosis of attention deficit disorder (ADD)/attention deficit hyperactivity disorder (ADHD) and to be more vulnerable, as a group, to respond impulsively to interpersonal challenges. One potential strategy that has received attention is targeting some of the known early risk factors for suicidal behaviors by using an upstream approach to suicide prevention with elementary-aged children. The PAX Good Behavior Game (GBG) is a classroom-based behavior management strategy that targets aggressive and disruptive behavior. Even though it was not developed as a suicide prevention program, it has been associated with a 50% reduction of risk for suicidal ideation and attempts by young adulthood (Wilcox et al., 2008). The PAX GBG is an evidence-based practice that is recommended by the Substance Abuse and Mental Health Service Administration, the Washington State Institute for Public Policy, and the Institute of Medicine. We have been very impressed with the work that is being done at our local schools using this approach. More information is available at https://www.goodbehaviorgame.org.

Black Girls Need Attention Too. Because Black girls have low numbers of suicide deaths, it may be tempting to dismiss this group as not at high risk and therefore not a high priority in suicide prevention programming. This is a mistake. In fact, the number of deaths among Black girls continues to escalate. The actual numbers are still relatively small, but the rates are increasing dramatically. Perhaps more alarming, however, is that the number of serious attempts among Black girls is extremely high. Almost 19% of Black high school girls made a suicide plan within the last year, and 12.5% had an attempt, which is the highest of any racial or ethnic category (CDC, 2018).

In interviews with Black female adolescents who had a suicide attempt, more than two-thirds say that they never intended to die. They make comments such as "I only wanted help. I didn't want to die" or "I knew that the method I used wasn't going to kill me." These stories give us insight into the mind of the Black adolescent female. They do not know how to reach out for help. One theory that has been put forward is that there is so much pressure on Black females to be strong and independent (called the strong Black woman [SBW] stereotype) that there is actually a negative effect on the mental health of young Black girls. They feel guilty or ashamed if they do not measure up to the perceived standard.

> *Practical strategy (schools and parents): Help Black females rede-fine SBW to <u>include</u> help seeking (e.g., "Strong Black women ask for support. When I ask for support, it is because I recognize that I am worthy of receiving help"). This strategy clearly will take a commu-nity and systems approach. The first step might be to ask impor-tant stakeholders to look at existing programming and messaging to determine whether the messages being sent are inadvertently contributing to the "go it alone" approach when it comes to mental health.*

Discrimination Is an Additive Risk Factor. Regardless of any other risk factors, experiencing discrimination raises the risk for suicidal ideation among Black youth. This is hardly surprising, given that discrimination has been linked to stress, low self-esteem, and depression, and experiencing discrimination as a young person has been linked to the deterioration of mental health decades later (Assari et al., 2017).

Black youth report spending more time online than their same-aged peers, and there are deepening concerns about the types of race-based discrimination that they face when they are online. For example, they may encounter racial messages directed specifically at them or threatening them, or vicarious racism, such as people saying things or making jokes or comments about their race. Black youth who complete daily logs now report that they have *more than five experiences of overt discrimination per day,* and the Internet is by far the most frequent context for the discrimination to occur. This is important, because previous research about discrimination with Black youth was all based on research that stated that discrimination with Black youth occurs about once per year (English et al., 2020). Clearly, the frequency with which Black adolescents face discrimination and racism helps contextualize the link between discrimination and suicide.

Practical strategy (schools): As the Black Lives Matter movement took hold across the country in 2020, one of the lessons that came from this movement was the importance of helping schools integrate essential and developmentally appropriate discussions into the classrooms. Crucial conversations about racism, discrimination, violence, and racial justice must be part of the living curriculum, not simply a stagnant lesson during Black History month. Uncomfortable conversations like these can lead to transformative learning for everyone in the school, creating a climate that promotes healthier spaces for African American/Black students and a better understanding for all students about how words and actions affect all members of the school community. Contextualizing these conversations within the restrictions that many states and localities have about critical race theory (CRT) can be challenging, but finding ways to uplift Black voices and experiences is important.

Latinx Students, Particularly Girls, Are at Elevated Risk for Suicide Attempts

Latinx students are more likely than their White peers to have unmet mental health needs, due to both cultural beliefs about mental health (stigma) and lack of access to mental health care. Culturally, there may be divisions between parents and children in beliefs about mental health, and religious sanctions against suicide may make talking about suicide particularly difficult for many within the Latinx community. There are also very real structural barriers to overcome. Latinx children make up 40% of the uninsured youth in the United States, even though they make up only 25% of the U.S. population. Additional barriers for some, such as language barriers, transportation problems, and, for those who are undocumented, the very real and present fear of deportation when interacting with anyone in a position of perceived authority, make it easy to understand why so many Latinx children are "falling through the cracks." For the Latinx children who *do* receive mental health care, 56% receive that care from their schools (Price & Khubchandani, 2019). It is for this reason that this population was particularly hard hit when schools moved to virtual learning during the 2020 pandemic.

Historically, Latinx adolescents have had high rates of suicide attempts, second only to AI/AN youth. Latinx youth also think about suicide at very high rates (girls more than twice as high as boys), and Latina youth have the highest rates of any group reported by the CDC of "feeling sad or hopeless." In fact, nearly 47% of Latinas report that they felt so sad or hopeless for at least a 2-week period during the last year that they stopped doing at least some of their usual activities (CDC, 2019). That rate is more than twice as high as for Latinos, and higher than for any other racial or ethnic group in the school. When nearly half of the Latinas say they meet criteria for clinical depression each year, there is clearly a problem of epidemic proportions.

Practical strategy (schools): School-based health clinics are uniquely positioned to intervene to address the social and behavioral, as well as the physical, determinants of student health. In schools with extremely high-risk/high-need populations that are unable or unwilling to make use of community resources, schools become the only viable option to care for student well-being. One option is the development of partnerships with local universities. This strategy can provide an opportunity, for example, for student nurses and

student counselors to provide integrated and interprofessional serv-
ices to a high-risk, high-needs population with poor health literacy
(see Parke et al., 2018 for more details).

Anti-Immigrant Rhetoric Raises Anxiety and Hopelessness.
In recent years, the Latinx community has faced higher rates of violence, discrimination, oppression, and racism as well as a national
wave of anti-immigrant rhetoric. More and more Latinx youth are
feeling the effects of these negative portrayals. In discussions with
Latinx children, they repeatedly make comments such as "We keep
hearing that they are going to keep us out. We know they don't want
us here. It makes us feel like we are no good."

In addition to the rhetoric, there are very real actions taken to
separate families and deport those who are not U.S. citizens or
who have come to the United States without proper documentation. For many Latinx children and adolescents, these actions have
made them feel more fearful and anxious. We have found that even
Latinx children who are documented might feel unsafe, not just for
themselves, but for their family members and for members of their
community. In an ethnic group already at risk for depression and
suicidal behaviors, the result has been even greater risk.

Religion May Play a Role, but It's Complicated. For years,
there was a strong belief that the role that religion played within
the Latinx community served as a protective factor for suicide.
The answer, however, may be a bit more complicated. For some
Latinx youth, religiosity may be beneficial, either because of the
connection to a higher power or because of the sense of belonging
and connectedness to a faith-based community. However, religion can also have a detrimental effect. There are those who believe that mental illness is caused by sin or lack of faith or that it
can be treated through prayer alone. Latinx children who come
from families who hold these beliefs are taught to feel shame or
embarrassment for their mental health problems and are discouraged from seeking help outside the family or from clergy. In these

instances, Latinx students may be left without a supportive adult to discuss their thoughts of suicide.

> *Practical strategy (schools): Helping families connect to faith-based counseling organizations can be a powerful way to reduce the stigma of mental health help seeking for those who have been reluctant see seek help because of strongly held religious beliefs. Schools can provide resources or opportunities for these faith-based organizations to provide presentations to help make the help-seeking process and the biological causes of mental illnesses more transparent.*

White Students Are the Most Likely to Die by Suicide, in Numbers of Deaths

For all that you have read and learned so far about the risk for suicide death among the different racial and ethnic groups, most adolescent suicide deaths have historically been, and continue to be, by White students, specifically White boys. Yes, the rates are higher for other populations, and yes, the rates are increasing among still others. But overall, in the United States, more than 80% of youth ages 15–24 who die by suicide are White, and more than two-thirds who die are White boys.

Much of the suicide prevention and intervention models and strategies that have been developed in the past have been criticized because they have used a "White-normative" approach. We *caution you strongly against* using models that have not been empirically tested on diverse samples or, more specifically, on samples that do not match the demographics of the students with whom you plan to use them. The critical message of this statistic, however, is that just because something has been demonstrated to work with White students does not mean it is not worth using. In fact, it may be perfectly appropriate for White students, who are, in fact, at risk. It just may not be appropriate for *all* students. And, if you have gotten this far into the chapter, it ought to be *abundantly clear* that when it comes to suicide prevention and intervention, *there is simply no one-size-fits-all approach*. Suicide prevention and intervention strategies will require many different approaches for many different types of students and their families. Knowing what works for whom (or what is most likely to work for whom) will give you a starting place for your work with the students, parents, teachers, and staff in your specific school building or district.

Age and Grade Level

Suicide remains relatively uncommon in young children (before age 10), although it certainly does exist. There is evidence that children as young as 5 years old die by suicide. Until recently, many people believed that young children couldn't die by suicide because they didn't have an adequate understanding of the finality of death. In our work, we have talked with *very young* children (ages 6 and 7) who have had extremely serious suicide attempts (jumps from buildings/bridges) who have most certainly understood what they were doing. This is consistent with newer research, and it may be that young children are now more exposed to advanced concepts of death, dying, and suicide than they were in the past. For whatever reason, researchers now believe that young children can, in fact, be suicidal.

In general, children under the age of 12 who die by suicide are more likely to have problems with family or friends, more likely to have higher rates of ADHD, and less likely to have a diagnosable mental illness, such as depression, than adolescents who die by suicide. This means that young children have more impulsive suicides. That certainly fits with our experience. It probably fits with your experience working with young children too. They simply are less planful than older children. Because we will discuss differences in prevention programming and intervention strategies by school level in later chapters in this text, we won't go into further detail here. For now, it may be sufficient to say that not only are there differences in suicide deaths but also there are differences in suicide ideation and behaviors, including how those manifest in thoughts and behaviors among young people in elementary, middle, and high school. Students in different grade levels require different types of interventions and programming based on their developmental levels.

Conclusion

Students in all demographic categories, of both sexes, as well as students who are transgender and gender fluid, of all sexual orientations, and of all races, ethnicities, and ages, can be at risk for suicide, although specific risk can vary. In general, boys complete suicide at higher rates than girls, even though girls engage in suicidal thoughts and behaviors at higher rates. Trans and gender nonbinary students are at even higher risk, as are students who identify as lesbian, gay, bisexual, or queer/questioning. Although most young people who die by suicide are White (in fact, are White boys), students of AI/AN descent or Asian American/Pacific Islanders have higher rates of suicide. Black students and Latinx students have historically lower rates of death, but rates are increasing dramatically among these populations.

Understanding the specific risks within each of these groups can help school personnel begin to create appropriate suicide prevention programming for their schools, and we always suggest that prevention programming start with this big-picture approach. However, an important take-home message from this chapter is that it is essential for school personnel to understand the students within their school and the risk factors for their specific population. Clearly, it is worth remembering that even once we understand the overall risk of certain populations, there is much variability within these larger groups, and this is where we turn our attention next. In the next chapter, we turn to a discussion of the most common *individual student risk* factors.

References

Assari, S., Lankarani, M. M., & Caldwell, C. H. (2017). Discrimination increases suicidal ideation in Black adolescents regardless of ethnicity and gender. *Behavioral Sciences, 7*, 1–10. doi:10.3390/bs7040075

Auerbach, R. P., Stewart, J. G., & Johnson, S. L. (2017). Impulsivity and suicidality in adolescent inpatients. *Journal of Abnormal Child Psychology, 45*(1), 91–103. doi: 10.1007/s10802-016-0146-8

Bichell, R. E. (2016, April 22). Suicide rates climb in U.S., particularly among adolescent girls. *NPR*. http://www.npr.org/sections/health-shots/2016/04/22/474888854/suicide-rates-climb-in-u-s-especially-among-adolescent-girls

Blashill, A. H., & Calzo, J. P. (2019). Sexual minority children: Mood disorders and suicidality disparities. *Journal of Affective Disorders, 246*, 96–98.

Brannon, R. (1985). A scale for measuring attitudes and masculinity. In A. Sargent (Ed.), *Beyond sex roles* (pp. 110–116). West.

Calzo, J. P. Poteat, V. P., Yochikawa, H., Russell, S. T., & Bogart, L. M. (2020). Person-environment fit and positive youth development in the context of high school gay-straight alliances. *Journal of Research on Adolescence, 30*(S1), 158–179. doi:10.1111/jora.12456

Centers for Disease Control and Prevention. (2017). Y*outh risk behavior survey: Data summary and trends report, 2007–2017.* U.S. Department of Health and Human Services.

Centers for Disease Control and Prevention. (2018a). National Vital Statistics System. *Mortality, 2017.* https://www.cdc.gov/nchs/fastats/suicide.htm

Centers for Disease Control and Prevention. (2018b). Suicide rates in the United States continue to increase. *NCHS Data Brief, no. 309.* National Center for Health Statistics.

Centers for Disease Control and Prevention. (2019). *Suicide ideation and behaviors among high school students—Youth Risk Behavior Survey—United States, 2019.* U.S. Department of Health and Human Services.

Choi, Y., Park, M., Lee, J. P., Yasui, M., & Kim, T. Y. (2018). Explicating acculturation strategies among Asian American youth: Subtypes and correlates across Filipino and Korean Americans. *Journal of Youth and Adolescents, 47*(10), 2818–2205. doi:10.1007/s10964-018-0862-1

Drapeau, C. W., & McIntosh, J. L. (2021, December 24). *U.S.A. suicide: 2020 Official final data*. Suicide Awareness Voices of Education (SAVE). https://save.org/wp-content/uploads/2022/01/2020datapgsv1a.pdf

Duong, J., & Bradshaw, C. (2014). Associations between bullying and engaging in aggressive and suicidal behaviors among sexual minority youth: The moderating role of connectiveness. *Journal of School Health, 84*(10), 636–645.

English, D., Lambert, S. F., Tynes, B. M., Bowleg, L., Zea, M. C., & Howard, L. C. (2020). Daily multidimensional racial discrimination among Black U.S. American adolescents. *Journal of Applied Developmental Psychology, 66*, 10168. doi:10.1016/j.appdev.2019.101068

Goodenow, C., Szalacha, L., & Westheimer, K. (2006). School support groups, other school factors, and the safety of sexual minority adolescents. *Psychology in the Schools, 43*, 573–589.

Gruberg, S., & Medina, C. (2022). *The 2022 legislative landscape for LGBTQI rights*. https://www.americanprogress.org/article/the-2022-legislative-landscape-for-lgbtqi-rights/

Haas, A. P., Eliason, M., Mays, V. M., Mathy, R. M., Cochran, S. D., D'Augelli, A. R. Silverman, M. M., Fisher, P. W., Hughes, T., Rosario, M., Russell, S. T., Malley, E., Reed, J., Litts, D. A., Haller, E., Sell, R. L., Remafedi, G., Bradford, J., Beautrais, A. L., Brown, G. K., Diamond, G. M., Friedman, M. S., Garafalo, R., Turner, M. S., Hollibaugh. A., & Clayton, P. J. (2010). Suicide and suicide risk in lesbian, gay, bisexual, and transgender populations: Review and recommendations, *Journal of Homosexuality, 58*(1), 10–51, DOI: 10.1080/00918369.2011.534038

Hatchel, T., Ingram, K. M., Mintz, S., Hartley, C., Valido, A., Espelage, D. L., & Wyman, P. (2019). Predictors of suicidal ideation and attempts among LGBTQ adolescents: The roles of help-seeking beliefs, peer victimization, depressive symptoms, and drug use. *Journal of Child and Family Studies, 28*, 2443–2455. doi:10.1007/s10826-019-01339-2

Hatzenbuehler, M. L., Birkett, M., Van Wagenen, A., & Meyer, I. H. (2014). Protective school climates and reduced risk for suicide ideation in sexual minority youth. *American Journal of Public Health, 104*(2), 279–286.

Juvrud, J., & Rennels, J. L. (2017). "I Don't Need Help": Gender differences in how gender stereotypes predict help-seeking. *Sex Roles, 76*, 27–39.

Kim, J. (2018). Beyond the trigger: The mental health consequences of in-home firearm access among children of gun owners. *Social Science and Medicine, 302*, 51–59. doi:10.1016/j.socscimed.2017.11.044

Kim, S. Y., Wang, Y., Deng, S., Alverez, R., & Li, J. (2011). Accent, perpetual foreigner stereotype, and perceived discrimination as indirect links between English proficiency and depressive symptoms in Chinese American adolescents. *Developmental Psychology, 47*(1), 289–301.

Mental Health America. (2018). *The state of mental health in America, 2019.* Author.

Musci, R. J., Hart, S. R., Ballard, E. D., Newcomer, A., Van Eck, K., Ialongo, N., & Wilcox, H. (2016). Trajectories of suicidal ideation from sixth through tenth grades in predicting suicide attempts in young adulthood in an urban African American cohort. *Suicide and Life-Threatening Behavior, 46*(3), 255–265.

Parke, K. A., Meireles, C. L., & Sickora, C. (2018). A nurse-led model of care to address social and behavioral determinants of health at a school-based health center. *Journal of School Health, 89*(5), 423–426.

Price, J. H., & Khubchandani, J. (2019). The changing characteristics of African-American adolescent suicides, 2001–2017. *Journal of Community Health, 44,* 756–763. doi:10.1007/s10900-019-00678-x

Qiao, N., & Bell, T. M. (2017). Indigenous adolescents' suicidal behaviors and risk factors: Evidence from the National Youth Risk Behavior Survey. *Journal of Immigrant Minority Health, 19,* 590–597. doi:10.1007/s10903-016-0443-x

Racine, N., McArthur, B. A., Cooke, J. E., Eirich, R., Zhu, J., & Madigan, S. (2021). Global prevalence of depressive and anxiety symptoms in children and adolescents during COVID-19: A meta-analysis. *JAMA Pediatrics, 175*(11), 1142–1150. doi:10.1001/jamapediatrics.2021.2482

Ream, G. (2019). What's unique about lesbian, gay, bisexual and transgender (LGBT) youth and young adult suicides? Findings from the National Violent Death Reporting System. *Journal of Adolescent Health, 64*(5), 602–607. doi:10.1016/j.jadohealth.2018.10.303

Reyes, H. L. M., Foshee, V. A., Niolon, P. H., Reidy, D. E., & Hall, J. E. (2016). Gender role attitudes and male adolescent dating violence perpetration: Normative beliefs as moderators. *Journal of Youth and Adolescence, 45*(2), 350–360. doi:10.1007/s10964-015-0278-0

Russell, S. T., Pollitt, A. M., Li, G., & Grossman, A. H. (2018). Chosen name use is linked to reduced depressive symptoms, suicidal ideation, and suicidal behavior among transgender youth. *Journal of Adolescent Health, 63*(4), 503–505. doi:10.1016/j.jadohealth.2018.02.003

Saewcy, E. M., Konishi, C., Rose, H. A., & Homma, Y. (2014). School-based strategies to reduce suicidal ideation, suicide attempts, and discrimination among sexual minority and heterosexual adolescents in Western Canada. *International Journal of Child, Youth and Family Studies, 1,* 89–112.

Toomey, R. B., Syvertsen, A. K., & Shramko, M. (2018). Transgender adolescent suicide behavior. *Pediatrics, 142*(4), e20174218. doi:10.1542/peds.2017-4218

Twenge, J. M., Joiner, T. E., Rogers, M L., & Martin, G. H. (2017). Increases in depressive symptoms, suicide-related outcomes, and suicide rates among U.S. adolescents after 2010 and links to increased new media screen time. *Clinical Psychological Science, 6*(1), 3–17. DOI: 10.1177/2167702617723376

Wahto R, Swift JK. (2016). Labels, gender-role conflict, stigma, and attitudes toward seeking psychological help in men. *American Journal of Mens Health, 10*(3):181–91. doi: 10.1177/1557988314561491.

Welford, J., & Powell, J. (2014). *A crisis in modern masculinity: Understanding the causes of male suicide.* CALM: Campaign Against Living Miserably.

Wilcox, H. C., Kellam, S. G., Brown, C. H., Poduska, J. M., Ialongo, N. S., Wang, W., & Anthony, J. C. (2008). The impact of two universal randomized first- and second-grade classroom interventions on young adult suicide ideation and attempts. *Drug and alcohol dependence, 95*, S60–S73.

YouthTruthSurvey.org. (2021). *Students weigh in: Part III: Learning and wellbeing during COVID-19.* https://youthtruthsurvey.org

3

Suicide in Context

What Places Students at Risk

Suicide is an extremely complex phenomenon. A dangerous pitfall people might make after a young person dies by suicide is looking for easy answers. Maybe it is our innate desire to try to make sense of something that can seem so senseless—but the answers to understanding suicide are never simple.

Our work with suicide prevention has brought us into contact with many parents who have lost children and with teachers or counselors who have lost students to suicide. We think about our work with a high school baseball coach who lost one of his students to suicide. The young man was sent home from baseball practice because he had a wad of chewing tobacco in his mouth, which violated school rules. When he arrived home in the middle of the afternoon, he found his father's gun and shot himself. Or we think of a local high school senior who killed himself the day the school posted up on the wall of the school the names of the colleges that all the seniors would be attending. He didn't get into the college of his choice, and everyone knew it. We work with a local volunteer for suicide prevention efforts who lost his daughter to suicide. She was a freshman in college when she called home to ask permission to use her parents' credit card to purchase a pizza. Her mother told her that they had already paid for the school's meal plan service, and she should eat at the cafeteria. The young woman killed herself later that evening.

These stories represent three terrible tragedies. But if we were to look only at the surface, it might be easy to get the wrong message.

Suicide and Self-Injury in Schools. Darcy Haag Granello, Paul F. Granello, Gerald A. Juhnke, Oxford University Press. © Oxford University Press 2023. DOI: 10.1093/oso/9780190059842.003.0003

Being sent home from baseball practice, facing your friends when they know you didn't get into the college of your choice, not getting to eat pizza for dinner—none of these was the reason behind the suicide. Each of these stories represents only the last little bit—the precipitating event, or the proverbial "straw that broke the camel's back." Each of these young people got to a place of suicide crisis through very different paths, and if we tell only this last little part of their stories, we fail to understand the true nature of suicide risk.

Everyone's pathway to a place of suicidal crisis is different. In this chapter, we will talk about some of the major suicide risk factors for children and adolescents. This can help us understand some of the major concerns that many suicidal students share. But these risk factors are useful only to the extent that they help us understand the overall problem of suicide and help schools create programming that meets the needs of the students most at risk. This is similar to the information in the last chapter, which helped us understand which groups of students are at highest risk. Knowing the groups that are at risk can help school personnel as they make decisions about prevention programming and intervention needs, but they can't predict which specific individual students will be at risk. It is with this cautionary note that we now turn to some of the most common risk factors for child and adolescent suicide.

To underscore the complexity of suicide risk, more than 75 different child and adolescent suicide risk factors have been identified in the literature (Granello, 2010). It is for this reason that we believe that simply creating lists of every risk factor ever identified is not very helpful for school personnel trying to figure out what to do. Therefore, only the most well-researched and -understood risk factors will be mentioned here, with the understanding that this is not a comprehensive listing. Of course, children and adolescents can exhibit some of these risk factors and not be suicidal. On the other hand, they can exhibit risks that have not been listed here and have thoughts of suicide or suicidal behaviors. The important thing for adults is to be aware of the risk factors, to know the resources available, and to be willing to have an open discussion with any student who may be at risk.

Suicide Risk Typically Comes From a Combination of Factors

Most people who study suicide now think about suicide risk in terms of a diathesis-stress model. That is, students have existing risks, predispositions, or vulnerabilities (the diathesis part of the model), such as mood disorders or cognitive impairments. Long-term negative life experiences, such as early-life adversities, poverty, abuse, or neglect, can also be thought of as a pre-existing vulnerability or diathesis. In the diathesis-stress model, these vulnerabilities are made worse by current stressors in the environment. From this perspective, it is important that the mental health professionals in the school building understand the lived experiences of students, including their past traumas and current mental health, to better contextualize each student's suicide risk. This lens also helps clarify why the current environment plays such a critical role in suicide risk. Students who are bullied, isolated, or discriminated against face current stressors (the stress part of the model). Taken together, how the brain responds to the current stressor can have a tremendous impact on how the student is able to manage the pre-existing suicide risk.

Importantly, the diathesis-stress model also helps us better understand the important role of protective factors for suicide. To the extent that resilience, coping skills, and self-esteem can help buffer some of the negative effects of stress (concepts that have been supported by research), enhancing these protective factors in the school curriculum may help lessen suicide risk (Kennedy et al., 2016; Timmons-Mitchell, 2017; Yen et al., 2015). *Nevertheless, schools must never send the message, either explicitly or implicitly, that students are responsible for meeting a hostile environment by simply having higher levels of resilience or mental toughness. Building up protective factors within students does not mean that bullying or intolerance is allowed to continue unchecked.* Rather, teaching young people healthy life skills that can contribute to positive mental health and enhanced coping, in spite of encounters with stressful or adverse life events, helps them understand that resilience is a dynamic and developmental process that takes place in all settings and throughout a lifetime (Suárez-Soto et al., 2019).

How Students' Pre-existing Vulnerabilities Contribute to Risk: The Role of Biology, Behavioral Disorders, and Unhealthy Thinking Patterns

We have all seen it—students who face incredibly challenging and stressful situations and seem to thrive while others face far less and seemingly fall apart. There are countless and complex reasons for these differences. At least one reason, however, is that some students have already had to overcome incredibly difficult challenges just to make it to school that day. They have faced so many difficulties in their young lives that their existing psychological resources are already tapped out. When they face new obstacles, they have nothing more to give. In this section, we turn to the internal (biological, cognitive, and personality-related) pre-existing risk factors that make at least some students more vulnerable to suicide.

Biological Risk: Depression, Anxiety, Impulsivity, Substance Use, and Sleep

About 20% of children and adolescents arrive at school each day with a diagnosed mental illness (usually a mood or anxiety disorder or attention deficit hyperactivity disorder [ADHD]), although many more meet criteria without a formal diagnosis or any type of treatment. These students have varying levels of risk for suicide, depending on level of severity and, of course, whether or not their disorder has been recognized and treated. It is quite clear that certain biological risk factors are associated with increases in suicidal thoughts and behaviors. However, we do not know with any certainty the precise role that any of these biological disorders play in suicide risk.

As an example of this complexity, consider the brain chemical serotonin, a chemical that we all commonly hear about that has clearly been linked to mood, most commonly to depression. There are studies linking serotonin levels to suicide risk, but it is probably not that simple (Oquendo et al., 2016). In fact, when looking at all of the available research, the combined effect of all the biological risk factors (not just serotonin, but all biological factors) on suicide risk is statistically significant, but not very practically significant. (For those of you who want the statistics, the predictive ability for combined biological factors produces a statistically significant but relatively weak odds ratio of 1:1.41 for suicide attempts, and for suicide deaths, an odds ratio of 1:1.18; Chang et al., 2016.) In other words, biology is only *slightly* able to predict suicide risk. If you stop and think about this, it is perhaps not surprising that the biological path to suicide is not that clear. Although many people who die by suicide have a mental disorder (most commonly depression, bipolar disorder, anxiety disorders, or schizophrenia), it is also clear that the vast majority of people with mental disorders *do not die by suicide.* In 2018, 25 million Americans had clinical depression. About 0.08% (or 8/100th of 1%) of them died by suicide. In other words, although biological factors clearly play a role, they cannot adequately explain who is at risk to attempt or die by suicide.

Depression Helps Predict Suicide in Students. Even though the pathway from depression to suicide is not a direct or linear one, decades of research, clinical practice, and interactions with suicidal youth underscore the importance of recognizing and treating depression. Depression is consistently recognized as a top risk factor for suicide, and this holds true across all ages, genders, and races among school-aged children (Ribeiro et al., 2018). Depression may have an internal cause (endogenous), but it is often caused by, or made worse by, external or environmental factors, such as bullying, poverty, or discrimination. Regardless of the cause, it requires recognition and attention. Left untreated, a depressive episode can last 6–9 months, which is an entire academic year.

Clinical depression can look different in children and adolescents than it does in adults. Although many depressed young people appear sad, hopeless, or blue, others can appear angry or irritable or act out in impulsive or aggressive ways. Children are also more likely to somaticize their depression (complain of stomachaches or headaches), and they may have disruptions in sleeping or eating. Symptoms such as feelings of worthlessness or guilt, excessive crying, or thoughts of suicide or death are also indicative of depression.

Practical strategy (schools): Unfortunately, people often use the word "depressed" when in fact they mean "sad." We hear students say things like "Our team lost. I'm so depressed." But clinical depression is not the same as sadness. When we use the term "depressed" instead of "sad," students who have felt sad and were able to pull themselves out of it (perhaps by going for a walk or talking to a friend) now believe that other students who say they are depressed should be able to feel better with these simple strategies too. More disturbingly, students with clinical depression start to believe that they should be able to simply feel better too. It is important to help students (and adults) differentiate between feeling sad and having depression. In classes, we often do this through role plays (for example, having students role play scenarios of sadness and depression, having the rest of the class guess which one it is, and then engaging in discussions of the differences and how friends could help). We are also extremely careful to be precise in our language and to help others use the correct term. To use the word "depressed" when we mean "sad" minimizes the lived experiences of those with clinical depression, with the potential for extremely negative outcomes.

The Role of Antidepressant Medication for Children and Adolescents. It is because of the very real danger that depression poses for children and adolescents that some of them are prescribed antidepressant medication. In 2004, the Food and Drug Administration (FDA) issued a black-box warning on antidepressants, indicating that they had been associated with an increased risk in suicidal thoughts and behaviors in some young people. This decision was based on the results of 24 clinical trials with more than 4,000 children and adolescents with a diagnosis of depression. The rate of suicidal thoughts or attempts was 3.8% for those who were prescribed a selective serotonin reuptake inhibitor (SSRI) versus 2.1% for those taking a placebo (Hammad et al., 2006). It is important to note that *no children in any of the studies actually died by suicide.* In more recent studies, researchers concluded that the benefits of antidepressants likely outweigh the risks to children and adolescents with major depression (and anxiety disorders; Bridge et al., 2007). The decision to issue a black-box warning was controversial at the time and remains so, as many believed it would keep parents from seeking appropriate medical care for their children. In the two years following the black-box warning, prescriptions of SSRIs for children and adolescents decreased by approximately 30% (Friedman, 2014). This occurred while the rate of suicides in this age group continued to rise.

It is not our place, nor the place of schools, to tell parents whether their children should be on antidepressants. However, we believe that an unintended consequence of the black-box warning was, and continues to be, to make some parents reluctant to seek appropriate care for their children. In 2007, the black-box warning was amended to state that depression itself increased the risk for suicide, with the hope that this would send the message that avoiding treatment was not the appropriate response.

It may be helpful to take a moment to understand something about how most people emerge from depressive episodes. Depression is a combination of negative thoughts, emotions, and behaviors, and these don't typically all improve at the same time. As students emerge from a depressive episode (this is true whether they are taking an SSRI or not), they usually regain their physical energy first, before their thinking and mood improves. In other words, as their energy improves, they have the energy to act on their suicidal thoughts. *Everyone* who is on an antidepressant should be monitored closely, particularly in the early stages of the medication. The increases in energy can trigger anxiety, agitation, and restlessness, which can be particularly dangerous while the suicidal thoughts remain. The available data suggests that there is a small but increased risk for suicidal ideation/attempts in the first 9 days after beginning treatment with SSRIs, although this increase is less than 1% and not statistically significant (Bridge et al., 2007). Nevertheless, when students are placed on antidepressant medication, the FDA has recommended weekly face-to-face follow-ups with the prescribing physician for the first 4 weeks, followed by monthly visits.

Practical strategy (schools): Adhering to best practices for the administration of psychotropic medication in schools is clearly important if school personnel will be handling these medications. However, even in instances when students will not be taking the medications during school hours, school staff are often asked to provide information to assist in deciding whether to place a student on medication and to provide feedback on the effectiveness or any potential side effects they may see. In the case of antidepressants, if parents inform appropriate school personnel when their children begin a course of antidepressants, members of the school staff can engage in heightened awareness and monitoring of the student.

Anxiety and Agitation Make Depression and Hopelessness Intolerable. Anxiety is the most common psychiatric disorder in children and adolescents, with as many as 25% of school-aged children meeting criteria for at least mild to moderate anxiety. There is ample evidence that rates of anxiety are increasing, as is the severity of symptoms. For years, suicidologists have been trying to understand the role that anxiety plays in suicidal thoughts and behaviors. Although anxiety disorders alone can elevate risk for suicide, it appears that the most significant and imminent danger comes when anxiety and depression occur together. When we describe this to parents or teachers who are trying to understand the mind of a suicidal student, we often talk about the student feeling depressed and hopeless and giving themselves negative self-messages. This is what Beck called the negative cognitive triad: negative view of self, of the world, and of the future (Beck, 1979). This might sound like: "I am a bad person (self)." "No one cares about me (world)." "It's never going to get any better (future)." Then, the anxiety comes along and pushes on that depression and hopelessness and says, "I have to do something about this *right now*; I cannot tolerate this for another moment." Depression and hopelessness make the student suicidal; anxiety makes the student feel pressured to act.

It also appears that social anxiety plays a role in loneliness and isolation, which are independent risk factors for suicide (Gallagher et al., 2014). Further, it may be that anxiety inhibits help seeking, which also contributes to risk. Whatever the mechanism behind the increased risk, it is clear that it is important to address the epidemic of anxiety within our schools.

Impulsivity Is a Particular Risk Among the Very Young. Children are far more likely than adults to have impulsive suicides. Children with high levels of impulsivity may have difficulty coping with stressful situations, may be aggressive, and could have ADHD. In fact, ADHD is the most common diagnosis among elementary-age children who die by suicide (Sheftall et al., 2016), although impulsivity remains a risk factor throughout adolescence (and, in fact, the remainder of the lifespan). It is easy to understand why impulsivity is such a risk, as it is characterized by immediate and unplanned actions (such as running into traffic or jumping out of a window).

There are some frightening clues about the high rates of impulsive suicides among the very young. Piecing together stories from young attempt survivors, we believe that about one-quarter of nearly lethal attempts occurred with *less than 5 minutes* between the decision to attempt suicide and the actual attempt, and as many as 85% of youth attempts occur within 3 hours of the decision. In other words, young people who attempt and die make the final decision and act upon it within minutes or hours (Bagge et al., 2013; Simon et al., 2001). *However,* it is important to note that even "impulsive" suicides do not come out of the blue. Rather, these suicides and suicide attempts occur in children and adolescents who are already at increased risk for suicide. For most, impulsivity refers to the final decision to act on the long-held thoughts.

Particularly among elementary- and even some middle-school-aged children, suicide appears to be a method for handling (or avoiding) interpersonal crisis and conflict. It appears that many of these young children do not necessarily have an underlying mental disorder, but simply do not have the interpersonal skills to handle difficult life situations.

It is for this reason that school-based suicide prevention strategies that focus only (or even primarily) on identifying and treating depression miss the mark, particularly for the youngest children.

Practical strategy (schools): Interpersonal problems are a triggering factor in many suicides among elementary school children. Therefore, teaching children skills in interpersonal problem-solving as well as building positive social and emotional regulation skills early in childhood may be an effective upstream approach to suicide prevention. In general, young children should be taught emotional identification and emotional expression. One intervention program that has been successful in improving emotional and interpersonal skills in young children is the Promoting Alternative Thinking Strategies program (PATHS), which provides instruction in the expression, understanding, and regulation of emotions (Greenberg et al., 1995).

Substances, Particularly Alcohol and Marijuana, Increase Risk in the Moment and Over Time. Adolescents who use and abuse substances are at increased risk for suicide. The two substances with the most clear and direct link to suicide are alcohol and marijuana. Teens who drink alcohol are at increased risk for suicide in the moment because alcohol decreases inhibition, increases impulsivity, and decreases problem-solving ability and rational thinking. Alcohol is also a central nervous system depressant, which can make depression worse. Long-term use of alcohol or marijuana by teenagers has been linked to increased risk for suicide. More frequent use of either of these substances has been linked to higher suicide risk, a finding that holds true across genders and across all racial groups.

We have a less clear understanding of how other substances (including opioids, cocaine, and amphetamines, among others) contribute to suicide risk. As an example, we have long known that teenagers who use tobacco are at increased risk for suicidal ideation. Of course, teenagers who smoke (or possibly use e-cigarettes, although this has not been well studied) could have other risk factors that contribute to this risk, such as lower levels of parental involvement. It also appears that adolescents who use opioids are at increased risk for suicide (Baiden et al., 2019), although clearly we will need more research as the opioid epidemic continues. Nevertheless, the important take-home message is that substance use and abuse places adolescents at risk for suicide, particularly if the youth have other vulnerabilities.

Insufficient Sleep Is Increasingly Being Linked to Depression, Hopelessness, and Suicide in Adolescents.   There is evidence that sufficient sleep is a protective factor for suicide. More and more, it has become apparent that adolescents, in particular, are chronically sleep deprived. Only about 9% of teens get the recommended 9 hours of sleep per night, and each hour of lost sleep is associated with a 38% increase in risk of feeling sad or hopeless and 58% increase in suicide attempts (Winsler et al., 2015). Lack of sleep also has been linked to increases in other high-risk behaviors, such as substance use and bullying. Importantly, it is not just quantity of sleep but also quality of sleep that matters. Sleep problems, such as nighttime awakenings and insomnia, *greatly increase* the risk for suicide attempts among adolescents (Koyawala et al., 2015).

Practical strategy (parents): Helping children develop good sleep hygiene is an important life skill that has many physical and mental health benefits. Some of the best strategies for children (and for adults too!) include (a) go to bed and get up at the same time every day; (b) put away phones and electronic devices late at night, as the blue light they emit stimulates cortisol, which tells the brain to be productive rather than to be restful; (c) exercise during the day to help our bodies be tired at night; and (d) avoid sugar and caffeine at night. It turns out that the timing of sleep matters too. We need rapid eye movement (REM) sleep to fully restore, and that most often occurs between 10 p.m. and 3 a.m. So, staying up until the wee hours of the morning and sleeping until noon on the weekends won't get teenagers the restorative REM sleep they need. Finally, parents serve as important role models. More than a third of U.S. adults say they sleep fewer than 6 hours per night.

Behavioral Disorders, Including Disruptive, Aggressive, and Risk-Taking Behaviors, Are Associated With Suicide Attempts. We don't fully understand why aggression increases suicide risk, but clearly aggression contributes to rejection by peers, which increases risk. It could also be that when young people respond to neutral situations with aggression, they are doing so because they have some basic cognitive distortions, which can ultimately increase suicide risk. Of course, aggression is also linked to higher alcohol and substance use.

Disruptive or aggressive behaviors in children and adolescents often go hand in hand with reckless or risk-taking behaviors that can lead to serious injury or death. Examples include driving under the influence, having unprotected sex, vandalism, interpersonal violence, and street racing. There are, of course, many other high-risk behaviors that are often part of the child and adolescent experiences. Sometimes, these behaviors are associated with underlying diagnoses, such as ADHD, oppositional defiant disorder, or conduct disorder. This is why youth involved with the juvenile justice system are at increased risk for suicide attempts. In other instances, these behaviors are associated with other pre-existing factors, such as low self-esteem, poor parental supervision, and school failure. Regardless of whether or not there is an underlying diagnosis, the focus in this section is on behaviors that are symptoms of internalized aggression or recklessness. When aggressive and risk-taking behaviors are part of a student's inherent makeup, they are clearly associated with elevated suicide risk.

Students also engage in reckless behavior because of peer pressure or social media challenges. Behaviors that are linked to social media are clearly different from underlying aggression and will be discussed in Chapter 4. It is also important to distinguish inherent aggression and reckless behaviors from nonsuicidal self-injury (such as cutting or burning), which also has been linked to increased suicide risk. Because of the risks associated with self-harm, there is an entire chapter within this book (Chapter 5) dedicated to the topic.

It sometimes surprises adults to hear that Russian roulette remains a significant problem among adolescents, sometimes with the added element of social media or YouTube, although YouTube has pledged to remove any such videos from its platform. Other high-risk behaviors demonstrate how recklessness and risk-taking can help desensitize students to death. As many as 1,000 young people in the United States (primarily males) die each year from autoerotic asphyxiation, which intentionally cuts off oxygen to the brain in order to intensify sexual arousal (Ibrahim et al., 2016). Various methods are used to achieve the level of oxygen depletion needed, although most people use strangulation or plastic bags over the head.

A Prior Suicide Attempt Increases Risk for a Future Attempt. Any student who has had a suicide attempt is at risk for another attempt. More than a quarter of adolescents who die have had a previous attempt. It could be that suicide attempts begin to desensitize people to the idea of hurting themselves. It could also be that students who are in the greatest distress simply have multiple attempts. Whatever the reason, it is important for school personnel to have appropriate plans in place for extra safeguards for any student who has had a previous suicide attempt.

Practical strategy (schools): Because of the high risk for a future attempt, students who return to school after a suicide attempt should have a "return to school support plan" in place that is designed to keep the student safe, supported, and connected. The details of these support plans are discussed in Chapter 9.

Unhealthy Thinking Patterns

Not all pre-existing vulnerabilities that elevate risk are biological in nature. Sometimes students have an increased risk for suicidal thoughts and behaviors because they are susceptible to certain patterns in their thinking. Of course, sometimes these patterns are caused by, or exacerbated by, biology (such as when depression feeds into hopelessness or when intellectual disabilities create rigid thinking). These patterns may also be the result of learned behaviors or basic temperament. Most likely these thinking patterns result from a combination of factors.

All-or-Nothing Thinking, Difficulties With Problem-Solving, and Overgeneralizations Heighten Risk. At least part of the increased risk comes from thinking patterns that are often associated with depression and suicide, including overgeneralization, catastrophizing, automatic thoughts, and all-or-nothing thinking. In other words, children and adolescents may think:

- "I failed this test. I am a failure. I will never be successful. I will fail at everything I try. I am a loser" (overgeneralization)
- "I didn't make the team. This is horrible. I can't bear it. What's the point? Life will never be good again." (catastrophizing)
- "I am a bad person. I don't deserve to be loved." (automatic thoughts)
- "How come I can't go to the pep rally? You *never* let me do *anything*." (all-or-nothing thinking)

There are other unproductive thought patterns that are worth identifying. This is important because much of the intervention work in suicide involves identifying, and appropriately challenging, the damaging and defeating thoughts that contribute to depression or suicidal thoughts. Not everyone in the school will be asked to play the role of challenging these thoughts with each individual student, but recognizing how they contribute to suicide risk is important for everyone involved to understand.

Practical strategy (self): Try to recognize (and maybe even keep track of) your own cognitive traps. Recognize what happens to your ability to problem-solve, generate options, and have hope for the future when you are stuck in these unproductive ways of thinking. As you consider the effects that these traps have on you, think about what you can do to help yourself recognize when they are occurring and work to challenge them. How can this exercise help you better understand the cognitive traps that may put children and adolescents at increased risk for suicide?

Hopelessness Makes Depression Feel Like It Will Last Forever. Hopelessness is an important risk factor in suicide, and it is the combination of depression and hopelessness that is particularly troubling. Remember, suicide is not about death. Students who are suicidal are in tremendous psychological pain. Edwin Schneidman, the "father of suicidology," called this pain "psych-ache"—a strong word to reflect the strong emotions and the severity of the pain. People who are hopeless believe that they will always feel this bad, and they cannot imagine enduring a lifetime of pain.

Perhaps you are already seeing the connection between hopelessness and those thinking patterns we just discussed. For example, if I fail at everything (overgeneralization), everything is terrible (catastrophizing), I never get to have any fun (all-or-nothing thinking), and I don't have any hope that any of this will ever change or get better (hopelessness), the path to suicide becomes a bit clearer.

Helplessness is related to hopelessness. When students are hopeless about the future, they can also become helpless, because they believe there is no way to take control and change the outcome. Helplessness, including learned helplessness, has been linked to suicide risk.

Poor Coping and Problem-Solving Skills Make It Difficult to Come Up With Healthy Alternatives. Young people, in general, have not yet developed the ability to engage in cognitively complex thinking. Children and adolescents tend to engage in more black-and-white thinking than adults, and as we already discussed, this type of thinking increases suicide risk. When they are in psychological pain and don't want to continue, they may decide that suicide is the way to make that pain go away. Once they come up with that "solution," they quit trying to find other ways to solve their problems. In one study, more than a third of adolescent attempters reported that they couldn't think of any other way to solve their problems (Esposito-Smythers et al., 2014). This is why it is so important to keep suicidal students from becoming isolated and, even more important, to make sure other people in their lives, including their peers, know how to help when a friend is feeling suicidal.

Practical strategy (schools): Students who are suicidal can become isolated rather quickly. This occurs because depression and hopelessness cause people to withdraw from others, and friends and peers tend to pull away from people who are depressed. The result is that when people are suicidal, there is no one around to challenge their all-or-nothing thinking or to help them problem-solve. This is why, when a suicidal student starts to think suicide is the only solution, it is extremely important that a friend or peer knows what to do, how to help, and how to offer other solutions (talk to a counselor, tell a parent, call the hotline). This is one of the best arguments for a school-wide universal approach to suicide prevention education.

Perfectionism Can Make Students Believe That They Aren't Good Enough. You may know stories of children or adolescents who appeared to have it all. They were good students, popular, and future oriented. When they were faced with a crisis, however, they were unable to cope. Perfectionism may be an even bigger risk factor among some children and adolescents than hopelessness (Smith et al., 2017).

Perfectionism can become like a broken record, repeating the internal message to students that they are not good enough, that they are a burden or a disappointment, and that they will never live up to others' (or their own) expectations. Then, perfectionism becomes an even greater risk because it makes it difficult for these same students to reach out to others and let them know that they are in distress or feeling suicidal, because they want to be seen as in control, free of flaws, and, well, perfect.

We have heard far too many stories of students who look like they have it all together who never received a suicide risk assessment because they didn't *seem* suicidal. It is easy to overlook these students who are suffering on the inside and smiling on the outside. We have too many sad stories: the cheerleader who was never asked, the young man with a full scholarship to a prestigious school, the articulate and outgoing child of a prominent local politician who worked on his father's campaign—we could go on, but the point is perhaps best made by one incredulous father who said to us, "She can't be suicidal. I bought her a horse!"

How Stressors From the Students' Environment Contribute to Risk: The Role of the Family, Adverse Childhood Experiences, Trauma, and Poverty

Of course, many students come to school with an elevated risk for suicide not because of innate biological, behavioral, or cognitive vulnerabilities but because of long-term negative life experiences. These have the same "diathesis" effect as biological vulnerabilities in the diathesis-stress model. Although these long-term experiences are complex and can escalate risk in many different ways, we will discuss just a few of the most relevant.

A Family History of Suicide Increases Risk for Attempts

Children and adolescents are more likely to attempt suicide if other members of their family have died by suicide in the past, with the highest risk occurring if the suicide was recent, especially within the past year (Kiriakidis, 2008). It is difficult to know whether this is due to biology, environment, or the effects of modeling. We know, for example, that young people who are exposed to suicide *in any form* (through school, friends, celebrity, media reports) can be at increased risk for copycat suicide, particularly if the aftermath of the suicide is handled poorly.

Of course, biology can help explain the increased risk among family members. There is ample evidence that certain mental disorders (e.g., depression, bipolar disorder, anxiety disorders, schizophrenia) run in families. However, biology alone cannot explain the elevated risk. Comparing all children with mood disorders, those who have lost a parent to suicide are 400% more likely to have a suicide attempt (Brent et al., 2015).

Family Dysfunction, Including Abuse and Trauma, Lead to Higher Rates of Depression, Hopelessness, and Suicide

Students who are maltreated, including those who are abused and neglected, are at increased risk for both suicidal ideation and behaviors. There are many different reasons, most of which are interconnected. For example, it is clear that in families where physical, sexual, and emotional abuse occurs, there are often many additional challenges, such as parental psychopathology, substance abuse, and neglect. Adolescents who experience abuse or neglect are also more likely to run away from home or experience homelessness (Ammerman et al., 2018). In addition, these students also often have higher rates of depression and hopelessness than those who do not report experiencing abuse or neglect. As just one example, children who experience sexual abuse are more than 3 times as likely as those who do not to have at least one suicide attempt by the time they reach early adulthood (Angelakis et al., 2019).

Exposure to trauma is also a significant risk factor for suicidal ideation and behavior. By its nature, trauma overwhelms the capacity to cope. Students who experience trauma can easily begin to believe that the world is a dangerous and out-of-control place. Whether or not the exposure to trauma leads to a diagnosis of posttraumatic stress disorder (PTSD), many of the most common reactions to trauma, such as anxiety, anger, hopelessness, and despair, can increase suicide risk. Other reactions, such losing trust in others, feeling threatened, or no longer believing in a higher being, can contribute to a sense of purposelessness. Some students who have experienced trauma and PTSD have told us that they now feel like a burden to those around them, and of course, that is a risk for suicide.

Practical strategy (schools): There are no easy answers to helping students who have experienced trauma within the school setting. Trauma-sensitive and trauma-informed schools are places where educators better understand the impact of trauma on student achievement and on overall behavior. In the case of suicide prevention, helping everyone in the building understand the link between trauma and suicide helps those interacting with students to do so with compassion and understanding, as well as with strategies to increase feelings of physical, social, and emotional safety. Trauma-informed schools increase access to behavioral and mental health services, collaborate with the community, and use positive and culturally responsive discipline policies. They are rooted in principles that (a) increase education for all staff about the impact of trauma on learning, (b) help students feel safe, (c) use a holistic approach to student physical and emotional well-being, (d) connect with community resources, (e) embrace accountability, and (f) anticipate and adapt to the ever-changing needs of students (nationalresilienceinstitute.org).

Students Living in Poverty Have Higher Rates of Suicide, but This May Be Due to Other Factors

Children and adolescents living in poverty have higher rates of suicide, particularly higher rates of death from firearms (Hoffman et al., 2019). However, children living in poverty also have higher rates of other challenges, such as family violence and social isolation, as well as lower access to mental health care. We find it fascinating that the elevated risk comes from the student's perspective of poverty, not from any objective measure of socioeconomic status (SES). In other words, students compare themselves to their peers and they decide whether they are rich, poor, or somewhere in between based on these comparisons. Once they decide where they stand, their beliefs about their own status appear to factor into their perceptions of their own worthiness and, ultimately, their beliefs about their own mental health. Students who believe they are poorer than their classmates are more likely to be depressed and suicidal.

One way to help improve mental health and lower suicide risk is to help students feel like they belong in the school. However, *this sense of belonging in school has only been found to be a protective factor among students with higher perceived subjective SES.* In other words, among students who already perceive that they are less well off than their peers, feeling like they belong to the school *has not yet been shown to reduce their suicide risk.* We want to be clear. This doesn't mean it won't help. It only means that students who perceive that they are already on the lowest rungs of their school are the most likely to think that their teachers and other adults in the school don't care about them or their learning and that they don't truly belong (Sampasa-Kanyinga & Hamilton, 2016).

Practical strategy (schools): Research shows that students in mental health distress who believe that they are of equal or higher SES than other kids in the school benefit from feeling connected to the school.

However, that same benefit of school connectedness has not been shown to improve mental health for the students who believe they are the poorest kids in the school. In this book, we try very hard to only give you the best practices based on research, whenever available. However, we are simply not willing to let this one go. We believe that those who see themselves as the poorest in the school often have extremely low self-worth. They may have more difficulty feeling connected. But this doesn't mean that schools shouldn't make concerted efforts to connect to them, even though we do not yet have strong empirical research to support these efforts. We hope that this research will come. In the meantime, the Centers for Disease Control and Prevention (CDC) has encouraged schools to think about connectedness in four main areas, and they remain the foundation of strong and healthy schools: (a) adult staff dedicating time, attention, and emotional support to students; (b) students belonging to positive and stable peer groups; (c) efforts to help students understand how school relates to their future goals; and (d) a positive school psychosocial climate (CDC, 2009).

Adverse Childhood Experiences, Which Measure Students' Accumulated Stress and Trauma, Are Associated With Elevated Suicide Risk

One way to understand the cumulative effects of a lifetime of toxic stress on suicide risk is through adverse childhood experiences (ACEs). ACEs harm children's brains so profoundly that the effects continue to be present years, and even decades, later. Hundreds of research studies have investigated the effects of high ACE scores on a multitude of physical, mental, and emotional disorders. ACE scores are determined by 10 items, including questions about experiencing physical, sexual, or verbal abuse; experiencing physical or emotional neglect; having a family member with a mental illness, substance abuse problem, or who has been imprisoned;

witnessing abuse of one's mother; and losing a parent to divorce, separation, or death.

Students with ACE scores of 3 or higher have rates of suicidal ideation or attempts that are 3 times higher than those with no ACEs (Thompson et al., 2018). Young people with ACE score of 7 or higher have a *51 times increase in suicide attempts*. In fact, *80% of all adolescent suicide attempts can be attributed to high ACE scores* (Dube et al., 2001). Although a lengthy discussion of ACE scores and what schools and communities can do to help build resilience in the face of students with high scores is beyond the scope of this book, we encourage everyone involved with youth suicide prevention and intervention to take time to investigate ACEs (see ACEsTooHigh.com to see the ACE instrument and to access the research on ACEs).

Practical strategy (schools): Go to the ACEsTooHigh.com website to investigate the 10 ACE that elevate suicide risk. Consider ways to determine average ACE scores or most common ACE for the students in your particular school to help understand how to tailor prevention and intervention strategies to your population.

How Current Stressors in the Students' Social Environment Can Contribute to Risk: The Role of Social Isolation, Peer Relationships, and Bullying

The biggest stressor (in the diathesis-stress model) for many students is their social environment. Peer connectedness and belonging are extremely important, and young people who either feel or actually are rejected by their peers are far more likely to report both suicidal thoughts and behaviors. During adolescence, as students become more and more attached to their peers (and less to their parents), peer relationships play an even bigger role in the determination of suicide risk.

Poor Peer Relationships, Peer Pressure, and the Breakup of Romantic Relationships All Contribute to Risk

Students who have poor peer relationships often also have poor social skills and low self-concept, which also contribute to suicide risk. Elementary-age students are more likely to report problems with friends as a risk for suicide, whereas teenagers tend to report problems in romantic relationships. Nevertheless, for all students, peer relationships and friendships are important, particularly as students begin to look more and more to their peers for support and validation.

Teens Themselves Say That Peer Pressure Plays a Large Role in Suicide Risk. Nearly three-fourths (73%) of teenagers say that teen suicides are caused more from peer pressure than from psychological problems (Debate.org, 2020). Although the reality of suicide is more complex than one singular cause, it speaks to the role that young people themselves believe that peer pressure plays in their lives. The need to feel connected, to be part of "what's in," and to be like everyone else, for some youth, can be stronger than the need to be well or the need to be themselves. At least for some students, peer pressure can lead to the fear of shame or embarrassment of not fitting in.

Practical strategy (schools): Using the power of peer pressure in a positive way is one of the reasons peer education campaigns, peer-to-peer educators, and other strategies designed by students, for students, to help prevent suicide are often seen as effective strategies. As an example, Ohio's Be Present Campaign is a social marketing campaign for youth, by youth (grounded in research, and with significant adult oversight and supervision), to allow students to lead the way in raising awareness about suicide and mental health, empowering their peers to take action, and taking more responsibility for helping each other. Campaigns such as these allow students, rather than adults, to take center stage in the development and implementation of social media campaigns, which give them a higher likelihood of acceptance by their peers (http://bepres entohio.org).

Isolation and Withdrawal Are Significant Risk Factors, and Loneliness Is a Term That Resonates With Young People

Isolation and withdrawal are suicide risk factors for all age groups but are particular risks for youth. The need for belonging begins in childhood but peaks in adolescence, where the necessity of belonging, of "fitting in," is so strong that social isolation can be devastating. Young people who start to withdraw (especially those who previously had strong social relationships) can be sending clear warning signs to others that they are at risk. We discussed earlier that withdrawal is often a symptom of depression. However, what we are hearing more and more is that even students who are still physically engaged with the world around them are responding to the word "lonely." When we ask if they are feeling alone, they point to the size of their online communities and the number of people physically present in their lives and perhaps say that they are not. However, when we ask if they are feeling "lonely," we are often overwhelmed with the degree to which this word resonates with their experience. More than 4 in 10 high school students say that they always feel lonely (Twenge et al., 2019), and upwards of 70% say that they often feel lonely. This probably isn't surprising. Current high school students are more likely than students from previous generations to spend their leisure time alone, connecting with other teens on their phones rather than getting together in person. We will discuss the seeming paradox that social media can create, with the appearance of closeness but with more time alone, in Chapter 4.

Practical strategy (parents): Parents can sometimes look at the lives of their adolescent children and mistake busyness for connectedness. They might believe that because there are many peers and "friends" in their child's life, their child is involved in many different social or after-school activities, or their child is "always on the phone," texting someone, or on the latest social media app, connecting to others, this means that loneliness isn't a problem. As adults, it is easy to believe that loneliness must look like depression, isolation, or withdrawal. Many young people, however, are fundamentally lonely and do not know how to tell others how they feel. One strategy might be to have the child take a "loneliness quiz" (the school might help by sending out a link to parents) that could be used to start a conversation between parent and child. Alternatively, parents and children together could brainstorm ideas (again, with the help of the school) to manage loneliness. Again, the most important aspect of this strategy is starting the conversation.

Practical strategy (schools): Many schools have felt pressure to cut their sports, art, music, and drama classes because of budget cuts or testing pressures. Yet these are some of the very opportunities within the school day that allow for socializing. Simply replacing these classes with after-school activities does not allow the most vulnerable students (those who have to work or who have families that cannot accommodate these schedules or afford associated fees) to participate. Rethinking these in-school social opportunities may be one more place to help lessen students' loneliness.

One strategy to help improve socialization that is receiving attention, particularly in middle schools, is assigned seating in the lunchroom. Mealtime has important social aspects. It is a time when we all develop social skills, and for most adults, food and socializing are linked. Yet many children do not have set dinnertimes at home to learn social skills, and for many lonely children with poor social skills, navigating the school cafeteria can be incredibly stressful. Schools that have implemented assigned seating strategies claim it helps students develop social skills as well as feel less lonely *and isolated. As an added benefit, these schools also claim that it decreases bullying behaviors.*

Loneliness and Isolation in a Postpandemic World.   During the 2020–2021 COVID pandemic and quarantine, the cumulative effects of school closures, the elimination of youth sports and school activities, and the cancellation of social events left children across the country feeling isolated, depressed, and anxious. Although studies on the long-term effects of the pandemic are not yet available, it is clear that few students have emerged from the lockdown unscathed. However, the 2020 quarantine was different from other types of adolescent isolation—it was imposed rather than self-initiated. It was also a universally shared event. These factors may offer a glimmer a hope.

Practical strategy (schools): Helping students make sense of their pandemic experience will be an ongoing challenge for schools. Every student will have this shared experience. Shaping their perspectives of it (was it terrible and isolating, was it scarring and depressing, or was it our generation's challenge that we overcame) can help frame how students will see the experience and perhaps use their time in isolation as something that becomes a generational connection.

Bullying

There is absolutely no doubt that kids who are bullied are more likely to think about suicide, have suicide attempts, and die by suicide. Students who are the perpetrators also are at higher risk for all of these outcomes. Kids who are bullied are more likely to be depressed and vulnerable to suicide, but vulnerable children and adolescents are also more likely to be the targets of chronic bullying (Klomek et al., 2019). Bullying becomes a cycle. Students might initially be singled out because they are different (perhaps they identify as LGBT or are a student with a disability), because they have few friends or poor social skills, or because others see that they already have some psychological struggles, such as depression or anxiety. When perpetrators of the bullying behaviors see that they had the intended effects of making their victims even more vulnerable, the bullying intensifies.

Bullying is remarkably common, and it is on the rise. In spite of all of the programming and efforts by many schools as well as large national campaigns to stop bullying, the number of students who said they were bullied at school within the last 30 days increased by 35% from 2016 to 2019 (Patchin & Hinduja, 2019), and 79.5% of students ages 12–17 say they have been bullied at school in a way that really affected their ability to learn (Hinduja & Patchin, 2017). Each day, 160,000 students stay home from school because of fear of bullying (David, 2016). Importantly, these numbers *do not include cyber-bullying*, a growing problem that we will discuss in the next chapter.

Unfortunately, the long-term effects of bullying can be profound. Victims are more likely to suffer from depression and low self-esteem well into adulthood. Students who observe the bullying in schools and see no one intervene are more likely to feel helpless and more likely to report thoughts of suicide (Rivers & Noret, 2013). Bullies themselves are more likely to engage in criminal behavior later in life. Although the link between bullying and suicide is complex, it is clear that being bullied or engaging in bullying behavior greatly increases suicide risk.

Practical strategy (schools): There are a lot of anti-bullying programs available for schools and a lot of pressure on schools to do something about the problem of bullying. However, in the rush to adopt an anti-bullying program, it is important to select a solid program with empirical evidence to support its effectiveness. For example, there was an influx of programming in the early 2000s intended to teach children how to intervene when a peer was being bullied. Although these programs seemed like a good idea and most of them stopped the bullying in the moment, follow-up research showed that many of them actually made the bullying worse in the long term. No one is sure why. It could be that the bullying simply resumed the next day, or it could be that the programs encouraged students to intervene in ways that were not natural to them, or perhaps students who had poor social skills were encouraged to intervene and they made the situation worse. The point is, schools must exercise caution when adopting any ready-made programming in their schools. When available, use programs that have solid research behind them, and be sure to monitor how effective the program is within your own school setting too.

Triggering Events: The Straw That Broke the Camel's Back

All of the risk factors in this chapter (as well as all the risk categories in the previous chapter) make students vulnerable to suicidal thoughts and behaviors. The underlying vulnerabilities (the diathesis in the diathesis-stress model) leave them psychologically depleted. The current stressors overwhelm them. Then, when something happens that pushes them past their ability to cope, they become suicidal. This is the suicidal trajectory. Looking to this last event, the suicidal reaction can appear out of proportion. Yet, when we understand the reaction in context, we see that they are responding to the entirety of the stressors that they are facing, not to the proverbial single straw.

In Students at Risk, There Is Often a Situation or Event That Pushes Them Past Their Capacity to Cope

Anything in a student's life could be considered a suicide-triggering event. There are two ways to look at this. First, if we remember that it is just the last in the series of stressors, we recognize that even a small stressor, piled onto the existing ones, can overwhelm the student's capacity to cope. But there is a second explanation that bears mentioning. Remember that adult and child perspectives about what constitutes a stressor are very different. When we talk to professionals about suicide risk in adolescents, we often ask them to think back to when they were young teenagers. Do you remember how serious everything seemed? How the reactions of friends meant everything? How a casual hello—or even a look—by a certain someone could make your day (and, conversely, a snub or rejection by that person could be the worst thing ever!)? Adults have more perspective and more experiences to draw upon, and are generally less emotion based in their behaviors. That is why well-meaning adults tell adolescents things like "there's other fish in the sea." From an adult perspective, we have all come to realize that the "love of our life" at age 13 will probably not end up being our life partner. But those types of comments are seldom helpful to the teenager involved. In fact, they can feel minimizing and dismissive and can end up making the situation worse (e.g., "Not only does the person I love ignore me, but my friends and family don't understand how terrible I feel! I am truly alone, and nobody cares!").

Remember, any situation can be a triggering event. Examples include the following:

- Any difficult transition (like the breakup of a romantic relationship, a parental divorce, a move to a new school, or graduation)
- A social embarrassment
- A conflict with friends, family, school officials, or the law
- The suicide of a family member, friend or classmate, or a celebrity
- The anniversary date of a significant trauma or painful life event
- An unwanted pregnancy
- Bullying, isolation, victimization

Most Students Demonstrate Clear Warning Signs That They Are Suicidal

Warning signs are specific behaviors suicidal students display that may help others recognize that they are at increased risk for suicide. Remember, the buildup to suicide usually takes time. For example, a typical path might be a student who has specific risk factors for suicide (e.g., depression, hopelessness, substance abuse), has one or more triggering conditions occur (e.g., breakup of relationship, legal involvement), and then demonstrates warning signs that indicate movement toward increased risk for suicide. Of course, not all suicidal individuals follow this path, but having a general idea of the progression toward elevated risk can be useful to help identify students at risk.

One of the clearest warning signs that a student can give is telling another person of their intent. More than 80% of adolescents who attempt or die by suicide tell another person of their plans. Other commonly occurring warning signs are as follows:

- Feeling hopeless, irritable, anxious, or severely depressed
- Engaging in aggressive, violent, or rebellious behavior
- Losing interest in activities once enjoyed
- Dwindling academic or school performance
- Withdrawing from friends, family, and relationships
- Feeling trapped, like there is no way out, or feeling "beyond help"
- Losing interest in hygiene, changing eating or sleeping habits
- Giving away prized possessions (Jason Foundation, 2022)

What is a consistent theme to all of these warning signs is that they represent a change from the student's previous level of functioning. Students may talk or write about death, for example, or engage in disruptive behavior, and others recognize that something is different. They realize that the current behavior simply doesn't seem like that person. That is the point. Warning signs tell us that something has changed. Most adolescents (more than 80%) demonstrate clear warning signs prior to their attempt or death. We have to make sure that everyone in the student's life recognizes these warning signs for what they are and knows how to intervene.

Conclusion

As we return to the stories that began the chapter, it is easy to see how the triggering events for each of these students could easily overshadow any underlying vulnerabilities that helped make them susceptible to suicide. Rather, using the diathesis-stress model, we must look at students with an understanding of risk factors (the diathesis) from an internal perspective (understanding the influences of biology, behavioral disorders, and thinking patterns), as well as the lens of the student's home environment (the role of family, ACEs, trauma, and poverty). We then add the students' current social environment (the stress in the model). Although there are different types of stressors, we focused on social isolation, peer relationships, and bullying. In the next chapter, we will turn to a very specific type of social stressor, the online world in which today's students spend so much time. It is within this complex interplay of biology and environment that for many students a triggering event occurs, and this becomes the proverbial "straw that broke the camel's back."

References

Ammerman, B. A., Serang, S., Jacobucci, R., Burke, T. A., Alloy, L. B., & McCloskey, M. S. (2018). Exploratory analysis of mediators of the relationship between childhood maltreatment and suicidal behavior. *Journal of Adolescence, 69,* 103–112.

Angelakis, I., Gillespie, E. M., & Panagioti, M. (2019). Childhood maltreatment and adult suicidality: A comprehensive systematic review with meta-analysis. *Psychological Medicine*, 1057–1058. doi:10.1017/S0033291718003823

Bagge, C. L., Littlefield, A. K., & Lee, H. J. (2013). Correlates of proximal premeditation among recently hospitalized suicide attempters. *Journal of Affective Disorders, 150*(2), 559–564.

Baiden, P., Graaf, G., Zaami, M., Acolatse, C. K., & Adeku, Y. (2019). Examining the association between prescription opioid misuse and suicidal behaviors among adolescent high school students in the United States. *Journal of psychiatric research, 112*, 44–51.

Beck, A. T. (1979). *Cognitive therapy of depression.* Guilford Press.

Brent, D. A., Melhem, N. M., Oquendo, M., Burke, A., Birmaher, B., Stanley, B., Biemesser, C., Keilp, J., Kolko, D., Ellis, S., Porta, G., Zelazny, J., Iyengar, S., & Mann, J. (2015). Familial pathways to early-onset suicide attempt: a 5.6-year prospective study. *JAMA psychiatry, 72*(2), 160–168.

Bridge, J. A., Iyengar, S., Salary, C. B., Barbe, R. P., Birmaher, B., & Pincus, H. A. (2007). Clinical response and risk for reported suicidal ideation and suicide attempts in pediatric antidepressant treatment: A meta-analysis of randomized controlled trials. *Journal of the American Medical Association, 297*, 1683–1696.

Centers for Disease Control and Prevention. (2009). *School connectedness: Strategies for increasing protective factors among youth.* U.S. Department of Health and Human Services.

Chang, B. P., Franklin, J. C., Ribeiro, J. D., Fox, K. R., Bentley, K. H., Kleiman, E. M., & Nock, M. K. (2016). Biological risk factors for suicidal behaviors: a meta-analysis. *Translational Psychiatry, 6*, e887; doi:10.1038/tp.2016.165

David-Ferdon, C., Vivolo-Kantor, A. M., Dahlberg, L. L., Marshall, K. J., Rainford, N. & Hall, J. E. (2016). A Comprehensive Technical Package for the Prevention of Youth Violence and Associated Risk Behaviors. Atlanta, GA: National Center for Injury Prevention and Control, Centers for Disease Control and Prevention.

Debate.org. (2020). *Are teen suicides more due to peer pressure (yes) or psychological problems (no)?* https://www.debate.org/opinions/are-teen-suicides-more-due-to-peer-pressure-yes-or-psychological-problems-no

Dube, S. R., Anda, R. F., Felitti, V. J., Chapman, D. P., Williamson, D. F., & Giles, W. H. (2001). Childhood abuse, household dysfunction, and the risk of attempted suicide throughout the life span: Findings from the Adverse Childhood Experiences study. *JAMA, 286*, 3089–3096. doi:10.1001/jama.286.24.3089

Esposito-Smythers, C., Weismoore, J., Zimmerman, R. P., Spirito, A. (2014). Suicidal behaviors among children and adolescents. In: Nock M. K., editor. *The Oxford handbook of suicide and self-injury.* New York, NY: Oxford University Press; 2014. pp. 61–81.

Friedman, R. A. (2014). Antidepressants' black box warning: 10 years later. *New England Journal of Medicine, 371,* 166–1668. doi:10.1056/NEJMp1408480

Gallagher, M., Prinstein, M.J., Simon, V. and Spirito, A. (2014). Social anxiety symptoms and suicidal ideation in a clinical sample of early adolescents: Examining loneliness and social support as longitudinal mediators. *Journal of Abnormal Child Psychology, 42,* 871–883. doi:org/10.1007/s10802-013-9844-7

Granello, D. H. (2010). The process of suicide risk assessment: Twelve core principles. *Journal of Counseling & Development, 88,* 363–371.

Greenberg, M. T., Kusche, C. A., Cook, E. T., & Quamma, J. P. (1995). Promoting emotional competence in school-aged children: The effects of the PATHS curriculum. *Developmental Psychopathology, 7*(1), 117–136.

Hammad, T. A., Laughren, T., & Racoosin, J. (2006). Suicidality in pediatric patients treated with antidepressant drugs. *Archives of General Psychiatry, 63,* 332–339.

Hinduja, S., & Patchin, J. W. (2017). Cultivating youth resilience to prevent bullying and cyberbullying victimization. *Child Abuse & Neglect, 73,* 51–62.

Hoffman, J. A., Stack, A. M., Samnaliey, M., Monuteauc, M. C., & Lee, L. K. (2019). Trends in visits and costs for mental health emergencies in a pediatric emergency department, 2010–2016. *Academy of Pediatrics, 19*(4), 386–393. doi:10.1016/j.acap.2019.02.006.

Ibrahim, A. P., Knipper, S. H., Brausch, A. M., & Thorne, E. K. (2016). Solitary participating in the "Choking Game" in Oregon. *Pediatrics, 138*(6), e20160778.

Kennedy, A., Cloutier, P. F., Gray, C., Cappelli, M., Ranney, M., Zemek, R., Jabbour, M., Reid, S., & Caldwell, W. (2016). Evaluation of a brief group intervention for adolescents with mild to moderate suicidal ideation: Building resilience and attachment in vulnerable adolescents. *Journal of the American Academy of Child & Adolescent Psychiatry, 55*(Supplement), S171–S172. doi:10.1016/j.jaac.2016.09.222.

Kiriakidis, S. P. (2008). Bullying and suicide attempts among adolescents kept in custody. *Crisis: The Journal of Crisis Intervention and Suicide Prevention, 29*(4), 216–218.

Klomek, A. B., Barzilay, S., Apter, A., Carli, V., Hoven, C. W., Sarchiapone, M., Hadlaczky, G., Balazs, J., Kereszteny, A., Brunner, R., Kaess, M., Bobes, J., Saiz, P. A., Cosman, D., Haring, C., Banzer, R., McMahon, E., Keeley, H., Kahn, J-P., . . . Wasserman, D. (2019). Bi-directional longitudinal associations between different types of bullying victimization, suicide ideation/attempts, and depression among a large sample of European adolescents. *Journal of Child Psychology and Psychiatry, 60*(2), 209–215.

Koyawala, N., Stevens, J., McBee-Straver, S. M., Cannon, E. A., & Bridge, J. A. (2015). Sleep problems and suicide attempts among adolescents: A case control study. *Behavioral Sleep Medicine, 13*(4), 285–295. doi:10.1080/15402002.2014.888655

National Resilience Institute. (2020). *6 ways to become a trauma informed school.* www.nationalresilienceinstitute.org

O'Carroll, P. W., Crosby, A., Mercy, J. A., Lee, R. K., & Simon, T. R. (2001). Interviewing suicide" decedents": a fourth strategy for risk factor assessment. *Suicide & Life-Threatening Behavior, 32,* 3.

Oquendo, M. A, Galfalvy, H., Sullivan, G. M., Miller, J. M., Milak, M. M., Sublette, M. E., Cisneros-Trujillo, S., Burke, A. K., Parsey, R. V., & Mann, J. (2016). Positron Emission Tomographic imaging of the serotonergic system and prediction of risk and lethality of future suicidal behavior. *Journal of the American Medical Association, Psychiatry, 73*(10), 1048–1055. doi:10.1001/jamapsychiatry.2016.1478

Patchin, J., & Hinduja, S. (2019). *School bullying rates increase by 35% from 2016 to 2019.* Cyberbullying Research Center. http://www.cyberbullying.org

Ribeiro, J. D., Huang, X., Fox, K. R., & Franklin, J. C. (2018). Depression and hopelessness as risk factors for suicide ideation, attempts, and death: Meta-analysis of longitudinal studies. *British Journal of Psychiatry, 212,* 279–286. doi:10.1192/bjp.2018.27

Rivers, I., & Noret, N. (2013). Potential suicide ideation and its association with observing bullying at school. *Journal of Adolescent Health, 23,* S32–S36.

Sampasa-Kanyinga, H., & Hamilton, H. A. (2016). Does socioeconomic status moderate the relationships between school connectedness with psychological distress, suicidal ideation and attempts in adolescents? *Preventive Medicine, 87,* 11–17.

Sheftall, A. H., Asti, L., Horowitz, L. M., Felts, A., Fontanella, C. A., Campo, J. V., & Bridge, J. A. (2016). Suicide in elementary school-aged children and early adolescents. *Pediatrics, 138*(4), e20160436. doi:10.1542/peds.2016-0436

Smith, M. M., Sherry, S. B., Chen, S., Saklofske, D. H., Mushquash, C., Flett, G. L., & Hewitt, P. L. (2017). The perniciousness of perfectionism: A meta-analytic review of the perfectionism–suicide relationship. *Journal of Personality, 86*(3), 522–542.

Suárez-Soto, E., Pereda, N., & Guilera, G. (2019). Poly-victimization, resilience, and suicidality among adolescents in child and youth-serving systems. *Children and Youth Services Review, 106,* 104500. doi:10.1016/j.childyouth.2019.104500

The Jason Foundation. (2022). *Suicide Risk Factors.* https://jasonfoundation.com/youth-suicide/risk-factors/

Thompson, M. P., Kingree, J. B., & Lamis, D. (2018). Associations of Adverse Childhood Experiences and suicidal behaviors in adulthood in a

U.S. nationally representative sample. *Child: Care, Health & Development*, *45*(1), 121–128. doi:10.1111/cch.12617

Timmons-Mitchell, J. (2017). Suicide prevention in community-based care: Evidence for the importance of resilience. *Journal of the American Academy of Child & Adolescent Psychiatry*, *56*(Supplement), S28. doi:10.1016/j.jaac.2017.07.800

Twenge, J. M., Spitzberg, B, H., & Campbell, W. K. (2019). Less in-person social interaction with peers among U.S. adolescents in the 21st century and links to loneliness. *Journal of Social and Personal Relationships, 36*, 1892–1913.

Winsler, A., Deutsch, A., Vorona, R. D., Payne, P. A., & Szklo-Coxe, M. (2015). Sleepless in Fairfax: The difference one more hour of sleep can make for teen hopelessness, suicidal ideation, and substance use. *Journal of Youth and Adolescence, 44*, 362–378. doi:10.1007/s10964-014-0170-3

Yen, C-F., Liu, T-L., Yang, P., & Hu, H-F. (2015). Risk and protective factors of suicidal ideation and attempts among adolescents with different types of school bullying involvement. *Archives of Suicide Research, 19*, 435–452. doi:10.1080/13811118.2015.1004490

4

Understanding How the Online World and Social Media Affect Suicide Risk

The Internet has transformed the way that children and adolescents learn and flourish, as well as ways in which they suffer, in ways that we don't fully understand. Schools are constantly adjusting to these new realities, as they help students use the Internet and the online world for the benefits of an almost endless supply of information and opportunities without falling into the many dangerous traps.

In this chapter, we will discuss some of the specific risks that the online world poses for children and adolescents in relation to suicide. Importantly, we will also offer some specific ways that schools can use digital connections to help prevent suicide. We recognize that wringing our hands and simply saying that we wish that our children wouldn't spend so much time on their phones or looking at computer screens probably isn't helpful. The genie is out of the bottle. We live in a world filled with virtual connections. Our students have only known a world with smartphones, computers, and social media. Our role is to teach them to understand and manage this technology in a way that helps them grow and thrive.

Suicide and Self-Injury in Schools. Darcy Haag Granello, Paul F. Granello, Gerald A. Juhnke,
Oxford University Press. © Oxford University Press 2023. DOI: 10.1093/oso/9780190059842.003.0004

The Pervasiveness of Technology in Students' Lives: Growing Up Online

Everywhere we look, we are surrounded by technology. Perhaps you are reading this chapter on some electronic device. At the very least, it is highly likely that your smartphone is neatly tucked by your side or next to you on your desk. You have probably checked it at least once since you started reading this chapter. Or, if you haven't done so yet, you probably will now that you have been prompted to do so! After all, it isn't just our children who are "addicted" to technology.

Students and Smartphones (or, "But Everyone Else Has One!")

If it seems as though every student in your school has a smartphone, you are probably correct. By 2018, more than 95% of high school students (97% of high school girls) had access to smartphones, a number that did not vary significantly by race, and varied only slightly by income (93% of teenagers with household incomes under $30,000 had access to smartphones, compared to 97% of teenagers living in households with incomes over $75,000; Statista.com, 2020). As parents wrestle with the decision about when children are old enough to have their own phone, more and more parents are coming to the conclusion that the "right" age is younger and younger. By 2019, for the first time, the majority of middle school children owned a cell phone. More than half of sixth graders (53%) and more than two-thirds of seventh graders (69%) had their own cell phone. As to be expected, cell phones are even making their way into the elementary grades. In 2019, nearly one in five third graders (19%) owned their own phone (Common Sense Media, 2019).

It is not just that more and more students have their own phones, of course, that makes school mental health professionals, administrators, teachers, and parents raise their eyebrows. It is a growing concern over how much time children spend on their phones and what they do on these devices once they are there. There is also growing concern over what all of this time on these devices might be doing to the mental health of students.

Daily Hours Spent Online Can Equate Nearly to a Full-Time Job, and More Hours Spent on Social Media Is Linked to Higher Suicidality.   A growing number of teenagers (nearly half in 2018) describe their own online use as "nearly constant." Elementary and middle school students (8–12-year-olds) spend an average of just under *5 hours a day* on screen media (not including screen use during school or for homework). High school students spend an average of *7½ hours a day* on screen media, again, not including screen use during school or for homework (Pew Research Center, 2018a).

There is no clear consensus about the general effects of all of this screen time. However, it appears that there may be some unintended consequences. Some researchers argue that overall, the use of electronic devices by today's youth is the single most important cause for higher rates of depression and anxiety among this generation (Hakoyama, 2019). Some point to the decline in face-to-face interactions among today's students as an example of the harmful effects of all of the screen time. As an example, the number of young people who say they spend time with their friends outside of school nearly every day dropped 40% from 2000 to 2015, with most of the decline coming since 2010. In general, the more time kids say they spend online, the less happy they say they are. Teenagers who spend more than 3 hours a day online are 35% more likely to have a suicide plan (Pew Research Center, 2018a).

During the 2020 pandemic and quarantine, many schoolchildren were forced to spend even more time online as schools moved to virtual formats and many parents, desperate to find ways to keep their children engaged when they could not leave the house, relaxed their limits on screen time. Experts struggled to give parents new screen time guidelines that were reasonable in what were unpredictable and uncertain times. What previously had been recommendations for a certain number of hours per day of screen time became "one media-free meal per day" or "two screen-free hours before bed." As families emerged from the pandemic and the changes to screen time routines it caused, they often found it was difficult to reimpose old rules and restrictions. What we have learned is that going back to the old ways may not be possible, or even optimal. What is clear is that it is important for parents, and schools, to develop new routines and new ways to manage screen time in a postpandemic world. It doesn't take long for students to question what they see as the hypocrisy to limits on screen time once parents, and schools, no longer have a need for young people to be online.

Practical strategy (parents): Limits on screen time for your child may be difficult, or nearly impossible, to enforce, particularly if they are teenagers. However, that doesn't mean that you can't encourage healthy screen time behaviors (and these tips are great for adults too!). For example:

- *Turn off automatic alerts, as these can encourage automatic behaviors.*
- *Limit (or eliminate) screen time in the evening—particularly during the 2 hours before bed.*
- *Engage in intermittent electronic fasting.*
- *Discourage the use of media entertainment during homework.*
- *Eliminate background TV. If no one is watching, turn it off.*
- *Keep screens out of your child's bedroom at night.*

- *Create tech-free zones (mealtime, or one evening a week).*
- *Limit your own screen time and model good online behavior.*

Schools also have a role to play in helping students understand the effects of screen time on their behavior and mental health. This means helping students manage the amount of time they are expected to be online, whether the school is operating in person or virtually. The pandemic offered many teachers and administrators the opportunity to structure online learning in ways that encouraged learning that didn't involve a screen. Although specific pedagogical strategies are beyond the scope of this book, it is important to remember that these choices can have significant mental health consequences for students.

Practical strategy (schools): When instruction is moved to an online format, schools must follow state and local requirements about number of instructional hours and what counts as "logged in." Some schools require live feeds with cameras on for instructional hours to count; others are more lenient. Most educators recognize that staring at computer screens for 6½ hours per day makes for difficult learning and contributes to poor mental health outcomes. Therefore, we encourage teachers, administrators, and school mental health professionals to be ever mindful of incorporating strategies to address student mental health within the confines of legal requirements. For example, scheduling physical breaks that include stretching and movement (or at least moving the eyes away from the screen) is important. Remember, in a traditional school building, students often walk between classes or physically move their bodies periodically throughout the day. Another strategy is to use "old fashioned" learning, like a paper and pencil (and then have students take a screen shot of their work that gets submitted electronically). Anything that keeps young eyes off of electronic screens can be one more way to help improve children's mental health.

Social Use of Smartphones Lowers Suicide Risk, but Overuse Is Linked to Higher Suicide Attempts . Smartphones are one of the most important ways that adolescents socialize. Notably, smartphone use for the purposes of socialization and outreach (defined as 1–2 hours per day) has been shown to be a protective factor against suicide attempts for teens (M-H. Kim et al., 2019). However, research shows that excessive smartphone use for young people is problematic. Teens who use their smartphones for more than 5 hours per day are significantly more likely to have suicide attempts (as well as increased depression, anxiety, stress, and low self-esteem). They also are more likely to have conflicts with their family members, problems at school, and difficult relationships with their peers, all of which contribute to poor mental health and elevated suicide risk. In addition, the more time teens spend on smartphones, the more likely they are to have poor social skills (Butt & Phillips, 2008), which is also a risk factor for poor mental health outcomes.

Of course, it's hard to say whether time spent on smartphones *causes* these interpersonal conflicts, mental health problems, and poor social skills or whether young people who are already feeling isolated and disengaged turn to technology at higher rates. However, there is some evidence that time spent on smartphones can reduce the quality of in-person relationships because interactions online diminish the capacity to recognize many social cues, including nonverbal ones (Bian & Leung, 2015). There is also evidence that addictive smartphone usage is related to impulsivity, and smartphone overuse can actually change brain physiology. In fact, smartphone overuse has been shown to decrease functional connectivity in the anterior insula and primary motor cortex (D. J. Kim et al., 2016), which alters the brain's ability to engage in higher executive function. In this way, cell phone overuse may be actually altering teens' developing brains in a way that puts them at higher risk for addiction, mood dysregulation, and impulsive behavior, including suicide.

Practical strategy (schools): Whether to allow students to have access to smartphones during school hours is a hotly debated topic, and school policies vary greatly from state to state and district to district. There clearly are pedagogical decisions that should come into play when making the decision about how to handle smartphones in schools. Our role, however, is to bring mental health and suicide prevention into the conversation. Again, there are no clear answers. Nevertheless, it is clear that students who do not have access to the latest technology may feel further ostracized if smartphones are permitted in class. Further, we have heard teachers comment that cell phones and earbuds are ways that students disengage from each other, which could squander opportunities for learning to engage and communicate with empathy. Regardless of the decisions that are made, keeping student mental health at the forefront of the discussions, and reassessing the effects of any decisions on student mental health, is important.

Screens and Teens: So Many Ways to Stay Connected

Of course, not all screen time is the same, and we are certainly not suggesting that all screen time has negative consequences for students. Clearly, there is important learning and valuable interpersonal connections that can take place in the online world. In the world of suicide prevention, there is ample evidence that highly suicidal individuals can find beneficial support, connections and belonging, and information that helps reduce their suicide risk online. We are great believers in using these online and social media tools to help do the important work of suicide prevention. But first we must gain a better understanding of what students are doing in their time spent online.

The specific sites, apps, and games that students use change with great frequency, and what is "in" today quickly becomes out of date.

We don't need to look any further than Facebook or email. By the time many adults were catching on to these methods of communication, many young people had long since moved on to newer ones. Similarly, YouTube, Instagram, Snapchat, or TikTok may be out of fashion by the time you read this chapter. The point is, regardless of the delivery platform, knowing how to help students make sense of their online experiences is essential.

Texts, Posts, and Blogs: When a Few Simple Words Can Spell Trouble

The need for teens to stay connected often starts with a few words typed into a tweet, an Instagram message, or instant messaging service, or a post to a chat room or blog. Sometimes, these quick posts turn into cyberbullying, which we will discuss later in this chapter. Sometimes, however, these messages contain cries for help or describe suicidal thoughts or plans. In our work, we often connect with students who tell us they learned of a peer's suicidal thoughts or behaviors from online discussions or postings. How these posts are received by others can make a difference and could very well save a child's life.

> *Practical strategy (schools): We believe it is essential that all students know what to do when they read a text, post, blog, or other online message from a friend or peer that threatens suicide or discusses suicidal plans. We have heard so many stories from students who told us after a suicide attempt or completion by a friend that they read something online but didn't know what to do or who to tell. Sometimes students are simply told to "tell an adult," but we have learned that (a) there is a fear among many students that this will be perceived as a betrayal by their friend and (b) many adults don't know what to do when given this information. Teaching students what to do when they read these messages takes time and education.*

Yes, young people clearly need to get adults involved, but adults need to be prepared to handle this information in a way that both helps the suicidal child and reinforces to the child who reported the information that this is the right, and safe, thing to do.

195 Reasons Why Digital Media Messaging Can Be Dangerous for Teens

Videos and electronic messaging are powerful ways to share information. Videos can capture our attention and our imagination by engaging our senses and luring us into the narrative. However, videos also have the potential to blur the line between reality and the digital world. It is for this reason that videos and media about suicide can be particularly risky to the adolescent mind, which does not yet have the capacity to cope with the intensity of the images. Even when the videos are not graphic in nature, it's clear that adolescents (and some adults!) have difficulty not getting caught up in a story and blurring the lines between what we see on screen and what is happening in our own lives.

In the 1990s, one of us (Darcy) conducted a study using a then-popular television show (*Beverly Hills, 90210*—the *first time* it was on television!), which makes this point. The show, a type of prime-time soap opera, was about a group of high school students in a wealthy community who go through an endless series of crises. When I interviewed a group of 12-year-old girls who watched the show, they essentially said they couldn't wait to reach high school, because they thought that the show modeled what high school life would be like. When I interviewed 16–17-year-olds, they said they wished they lived in California, because clearly high school was not like that for them *primarily because* they were living in a small town in Ohio. When I interviewed a group of 21-year-olds, they laughed at the naivete of younger girls who thought high school would be like the television show. They knew better. However, unprompted, they pointed to a newer series, *Melrose Place*, which was a prime-time soap opera that followed the lives of young adults. They looked to this show to help them understand the reality of young adulthood (Granello, 1997). The point of this is that all of the girls and young women in this study could tell me that they knew the television show was not real. *However, when they started discussing the show with one another, the lines blurred, and they forgot that it wasn't real.* That is the danger, and it is particularly troublesome when stories, images, and videos revolve around mental health and suicide. Children and adolescents who overidentify with the people or characters in the videos or shows can have trouble de-individuating from what and who they see online.

In 2017, Netflix released season 1 of a highly controversial show, *13 Reasons Why* (13RW), which chronicled the story of an adolescent girl who kills herself through a series of 13 recordings that she leaves behind for those she believes are to blame for her death. The show was both acclaimed by some as a way to present information about suicide to younger audiences and widely critiqued by suicide prevention experts over fears of contagion, simplistic messaging, and lack of adherence to reporting guidelines on suicide. In the weeks and months following its release, many argued that the show had increased call volumes to suicide hotlines, while others argued that the increased calls were evidence of greater awareness and help seeking. Bridge and his coauthors (2020) in the largest attempt to measure the effects of 13RW found that the release of the show in 2017 was responsible for 195 additional suicide deaths nationally among 10–17-year-olds, with most of these deaths occurring within 1 month after the release of the Netflix series, and the remaining occurring within the subsequent 2 months. In short, these additional deaths represent 195 reasons why schools need to pay attention to the digital messaging their students are consuming—and to give students the necessary skills to manage what they see online.

This overidentification extends beyond television. There is clear evidence that adolescents' suicide rates increase during the 2 weeks that follow media coverage of an adolescent's suicide, with overidentification with the person who died as the most commonly accepted explanation. There is also clear evidence that adolescent suicide rates increase in the 2 weeks following media coverage of a celebrity. This is why, in 2011, the American Foundation for Suicide Prevention developed specific guidelines for discussing suicide and reporting suicide deaths in the media. We will explain these in more detail in Chapter 10.

Practical strategy (schools): The same powerful reasons that help blur the lines between the digital world and reality in negative ways can help young viewers engage with positive messages and educational content about suicide prevention. There is reason to believe that people are seeking out these types of messages online. A study that analyzed teen suicide videos on YouTube, each with more than 1,000 views, found 413 videos with nearly half a billion cumulative views (Dagar & Falcone, 2020). They found that nearly half of these videos (49%) were educational and almost a third (30%) were about awareness/prevention. In other words, people are willing watch online videos (half a billion times!) to learn what they can do to help prevent suicide, and this has powerful implications for school-based suicide prevention programming. Using positive video messaging for suicide prevention programming can be a powerful strategy to engage students.

Social Media: Where Being Liked Does Not Equate to Being Loved

In 2017, the first large-scale study of its kind began to measure the effects of social media on teenagers (Twenge et al., 2017). The results were disturbing and caused many adults to change their perception of social media from simply a way for kids to communicate with their friends to something that had the potential to drastically harm their mental health. In general, the study found that adolescents who spent more time on social media were more likely to report significant mental health concerns and suicide-related outcomes. These negative outcomes were more pronounced among girls than boys.

Since that time, the effects of social media on the mental health of young people have been the focus of countless studies and endless debate and discussion, with very few clear answers. Here is what we know: excessive social media use is linked to higher rates of suicide and depression among girls, but it also can provide the opportunity for life-saving interventions, if posts reveal suicidal ideation or intent that prompt peers or parents to take action.

What causes the higher rates of depression and suicidal behaviors is less clear. It appears there are some particular aspects of social media itself that combine with both adolescent development and specific risks for suicide that come together to create a perfect storm. In other words, social media sites, as well as other technological giants, such as Google and YouTube, use sophisticated algorithms to manipulate the user and influence behavior, using complex psychological strategies to engage the user and control the content that they see. These algorithms distort reality, share misinformation, and disorient the user. That means that social media can be addictive and disorienting for people of all ages. However, social media is particularly appealing for adolescents, where it offers a way to amplify and accelerate the main developmental task of belongingness. More than anything, most young people want to fit in and find their identity through connections with peers, and these sites, with their inherent flaws, can become the primary method that teens use to accomplish the most important task of their young lives. When these social media sites inevitably do not allow them to meet their developmental needs, many young people are faced with dangers that fit neatly into Joiner's interpersonal theory of suicide. Joiner (2005) stated that thwarted belonging and perceived burdensomeness are two of the major factors that drive suicide.

When social media fails to offer the sense of belonging that young people crave (or, in many cases, offers outright social rejection) or when it creates a sense that others would be better off without them, social media can actually amplify depression, anxiety, and suicidal thoughts and behaviors.

In our work, we hear young people (particularly young girls) say things like "After hours of scrolling through my Instagram feeds, I just feel worse about myself." Even our graduate students admit that when they see posts from their friends online, it's hard not to compare their lives, or their looks, to the images online and feel bad.

Practical strategy (schools): It seems that girls are particularly susceptible to some of the negative consequences of extended time spent on social media, such as higher rates of envy, fear of missing out, and higher rates of negative self-evaluation, as well as lower rates of happiness, self-esteem, and life satisfaction. More time spent on social media has also been associated with higher rates of disordered eating in girls. Creating face-to-face opportunities for girls to socialize and engage in activities may be one way to help reduce the amount of time spent on social media, which could help lessen these negative effects. Although there is not a lot of research on the long-term effectiveness of these types of in-person school-based programs on reducing social media time, the research that does exist suggests that providing opportunities for before-school, noon-hour, or after-school intramural, noncompetitive, or competitive physical activity programs is associated with less screen-time use by teenage girls (Katapally et al., 2017).

Regardless of Online Platform, Teens Are Mixed About the Effects Social Media Has on Their Own Mental Health. Although they are spending a lot of time on social media, there is no clear consensus among young people about the effects it is having on their own mental health. Nearly half (45%) are uncertain if the effects of time on social media, overall, are positive or negative, while about a third (31%) believe that, in general, social media has a positive effect on people their age. The remaining 24%, however, believe that the overall effects of social media have mostly been negative on people their age (Pew Research Center, 2018a). The lack of consensus highlights the overall uncertainty that young people have about this very real, very large presence in their lives. We believe that this uncertainty also means that there is a space for adults to help them engage in more critical and thoughtful analysis of the material they read and of the experiences they have online.

Practical strategy (schools): As with most things, social media is probably neither "good" nor "bad." How, when, why, and by whom it is used, however, can certainly have positive or negative effects on the mental health of the users. Because schools are places for learning, they are ideal places for fact-based education and training about the use of this communication tool. In our experience, students complain that adults in their lives simply tell them that social media is bad or that they should put away their phones, or that schools only highlight the negative effects of social media. Of course, this approach is seldom useful and certainly doesn't encourage students to be thoughtful and intentional about incorporating the positive aspects of social media into their lives while making clear and deliberate plans to minimize the negative outcomes. Rather, treating social media as a communication tool, like any other, and teaching strategies for its use may have more productive outcomes.

The Scary Stuff: Cyberbullying, Social Media Challenges, and the Things That Keep Adults Up at Night

Okay, let's get the chilling and dangerous parts of technology out of the way first. If you are like most people reading this book, you won't be able to concentrate on the positive aspects of technology or think about how you can use social media to benefit young people until we talk about all the frightening scenarios you may have heard about: a live video stream of a young man's suicide on Facebook that later went viral on TikTok; a court case of a young woman who sent thousands of texts to her boyfriend, bullying him into suicide; a high school student who jumped off a bridge after he was catfished and then blackmailed on Skype; a 13-year-old who died after a topless selfie intended for her boyfriend was shared with her entire class; a middle schooler who hanged himself after he asked his parents to homeschool him because he was teased at school, only to have the teasing continue online. We could continue...

The Internet allows for heightened levels of aggression and intolerance toward others. There are several key reasons this occurs. First, an overarching principle from social psychology is that as group size increases, each individual's perceived responsibility for the group's actions decreases. In this case, the sheer enormity of the Internet means that each individual feels very little responsibility for incidents of cyberbullying committed by others, making it easier for each person to participate. Added to the lack of individual responsibility is a concept called deindividuation, or the concept that people act differently in crowds than they do individually. The anonymity of the Internet means that people no longer fear evaluation from others, but deindividuation also allows people to feel less self-aware, meaning that they do not tend to engage in negative self-evaluation either. Rather, they tend to simply follow the group's norms and behaviors. Others argue that social contagion means that each person's aggressive or impulsive tendencies are magnified in large crowds, causing them to act more violently or impulsively than they would if they were alone. Put together, the Internet is the "perfect storm" for escalating acts of cyberaggression. It also is a place where kids who are lonely, isolated, and impressionable can make poor decisions.

Cyberbullying

Cyberbullying is the use of any electronic device to "intimidate, threaten, or humiliate another" via text or images sent via the Internet or other forms of electronic communication (Kowalski et al., 2008). There are many different mechanisms through which young people engage in cyberbullying, but it is often through the use of embarrassing, offensive, degrading, or threatening text or instant messages; through the spreading of malicious rumors or the sharing of private information or images; or by masquerading as another person (often referred to as catfishing). Sometimes cyberbullying takes the form of the creation of graphic websites, images, or social networking site pages designed to harass or embarrass a person (e.g., ranking the "fattest" or "sluttiest" student; Cohen-Almagor, 2018). Although traditionally, the definition of face-to-face bullying typically involves an imbalance of power and repetition; these are not as clear for cyberbullying. In fact, although physical bullying typically involves an aggressor who is more physically powerful than a victim and often has more perceived power and status in the social circle in which both parties operate, these criteria are not necessarily true in the online format of cyberbullying. Further, although the cyberbullying itself may not be repetitive (although it often is), one single image or post can have ongoing effects. It can be posted on multiple sites, with lingering and painful effects for the victim. The scale and scope of cyberbullying, and the speed with which the information travels, is mind-numbing.

Finally, and perhaps most devastating of all, there is no escape. It occurs 24 hours a day, 7 days a week, over summer holidays and school vacations, on every electronic device, without refuge.

Practical strategy (schools): Keeping up with the ways that students engage in cyberbullying can feel like a full-time job. One website lists 42 different strategies that teens use to engage in cyberbullying (Nuccitelli, 2020), and even that is clearly not an exhaustive list.

Although it is impossible to keep up with every trend, it is worthwhile for school mental health personnel to be aware of some of the latest cyberbullying trends, especially those that are occurring within their schools. Here are some terms to get you started:

- *Bash boards—cyberbullying in chat rooms or message boards*
- *Catfishing—setting up a fictitious online profile to attract a victim into a romantic relationship*
- *Exclusion—ostracizing a child from certain events online, such as not allowing them into certain webpages or deleting their comments so they cannot be heard*
- *Flaming—getting into heated public arguments, usually with extreme profanity*
- *Griefing—irritating and angering people in video games by intentionally creating a destructive character*
- *Impersonation (imping)—impersonating the victim online and then saying embarrassing or mean things to create a bad impression of the victim to others*
- *Happy slapping—publishing embarrassing images or images of a victim being physically assaulted*
- *Outing—making public information that was shared privately, such as sharing information about a crush that someone has or information about someone's sexual orientation*
- *Phishing—tricking victims into sharing personal information*
- *Sextortion—threats to expose sexually explicit images unless a victim does something, in order to humiliate or seek revenge*
- *Slut shaming—a term used to criticize people, especially women, who violate the societal expectations of sexual behavior or appearance*
- *Trolling—intentionally antagonizing another person online by posting inflammatory or offensive comments about them*

Practical strategy (schools): Students should have very clear information about what to do if they, or someone they know, are the victim of cyberbullying. Although there are no clear answers to this growing societal problem, having a set policy in place that is clearly defined and readily available to students, parents, teachers, and administrators will make sure that these policies are enacted swiftly and equitably, and without regard to the individual personalities involved.

Cyberbullying and Suicide: The Combination of Cyberbullying and School-Based Bullying That Represents the Biggest Threat. Cyberbullying has real and lasting impacts on the mental health of children and teenagers. A 2020 study found that 44% of young people who were cyberbullied developed social anxiety, 36% developed depression, and a third (33%) said they had suicidal thoughts (Hackett, 2020). Yet when researchers spend more time with these numbers, they see a more complex picture. What they learn is that students who are only bullied at school OR who are only cyberbullied are only slightly more likely than students who are not bullied at all to think about suicide and no more likely than the nonbullied students to attempt to take their own lives (Hinduja & Patchin, 2018a; Patchin, 2018). However, students who are *both bullied at school and cyberbullied* are 5 times more likely to think about suicide and 11 times more likely to have a suicide attempt (Hinduja & Patchin, 2018a). In other words, when surveys ask students if they have been cyberbullied and if they are suicidal, they should be asking if they have been bullied face to face as well. It appears that students who face both these types of bullying are at the highest risk for suicidal thoughts and attempts.

Practical strategy (parents): Research shows that about 12% of parents (1 in 10) say that their child has been the victim of cyberbul-lying, yet a 2018 Pew Research Study found that 59% of teens report that they are cyberbullied each year (Pew Research Center, 2018b). The disconnect is clear—and troubling. Most parents respond pos-itively after they learn that their child has been cyberbullied (most

*often by talking with their child about Internet safety, adjusting pa-
rental controls to block offenders, saving evidence for investigators,
or talking with the child's school). However, if parents do not know
what is happening in their child's life, they cannot provide safety,
use the opportunity for learning, or watch for signs of plummeting
mental health. Helping their children understand the importance
of engaging in open conversations about any cyberbullying they
are experiencing is an important, if admittedly sometimes difficult,
first step. Once a parent learns of their child's cyberbullying, the first
and most important step is to make sure the child is (and feels) safe.
Other important steps (Hinduja & Patchin, 2018a) include the
following:*

- *Talk with (and listen to) your child.*
- *Collect evidence.*
- *Work with the school.*
- *Refrain from contacting the parents of the bully, as this could es-
  calate the problem.*
- *Seek counseling for your child, if appropriate.*
- *Contact the police, if necessary, to ensure safety.*
- *Implement procedures to keep it from happening again.*

Clearly, schools have an important role in the prevention of cyberbullying, even though many incidents occur off school premises and outside of normal school hours. Across the country school
buildings and districts have worked to develop policies to address
this growing crisis. Describing the details and nuances of all of these
different policies would be a massive undertaking and is clearly beyond the scope of this book. Nevertheless, we encourage all school
mental health personnel to take time to revisit their cyberbullying
policies and procedures to make sure they are up to date and in line
with current best practices.

*Practical strategy (schools): Each school building will have dif-
ferent specific policies regarding cyberbullying that fit their specific*

needs, the developmental level of their student body, and the state laws within which they operate. Nevertheless, there are some over-arching considerations, such as those outlined by Hinduja and Patchin (2018b), to consider when implementing or updating these policies (see Hinduja & Patchin, 2018b for a full listing):

- *Formally assess the extent of the problem by surveying your current students to get a baseline measure of the level of cyberbullying.*
- *Develop a clear protocol and policy about cyberbullying, including acceptable uses of electronic devices on school premises. Explain to students that cyberbullying is always unacceptable and explain why.*
- *Cultivate a positive school atmosphere that promotes connectiveness and respect.*
- *Develop and implement an established procedure for how cyberbul-lying will be handled once it becomes known.*
- *Assign a person who will become the cyberbullying expert for the building, keeping the policy up to date, keeping up with the latest research and ideas about cyberbullying, and sharing updates with others in the building.*

Social Media Challenges: Hunting the Elusive Blue Whale

Beginning in the summer of 2015, a new and frightening global trend began to emerge among children and adolescents. Suddenly, hundreds, and eventually thousands, of children, teenagers, and young adults around the globe downloaded the Blue Whale Challenge onto their electronic devices and began to follow the directives contained within the game (Jaitly et al., 2018). These tasks, given by the game's curators, required participants to send photos as proof that they had completed them and were committed to the Blue Whale. As the game continued, the tasks became more psy-chologically and physically damaging, eventually creating extreme psychological trauma in the game's participants, in preparation for the final command, which was to require participants to die by suicide. Early commands included:

- Wake up at 4:20 a.m. and watch psychedelic and scary videos that the curator sends you.
- Cut your arm with a razor along your veins, but not too deep.
- Poke your hand with a needle many times.

Eventually, the commands became more life threatening, including:

- Go to the highest roof and stand on the edge.
- Wake up at 4:20 a.m. and go to rails (train tracks).

The 50th and final command from the curator was simply:

- Jump off a high building. Take your life.

No one is sure how many people died as a direct result of the Blue Whale Challenge or how many young people participated in these directives. One study in India found that over 2,000 children had downloaded the game on their devices (Desk, 2017). Once parents became aware of the trend and started looking on their children's electronic devices, it became apparent that the Blue Whale Challenge was a significant problem.

There are other types of social media challenges, pro-suicide websites, and online games that promote suicide. For example, there was a Japanese message board that described a way to die using hydrogen sulfide gas. Within weeks, 220 people had attempted to die using this method, with 208 confirmed deaths (Luxton et al., 2012). There are several popular pro-suicide sites that have been directly linked to the death of children and adolescents, although in line with best practices, we will not name them here. We often talk with parents about Whisper.sh, an extremely popular website and app that allows young people to post their deepest secrets and then encourages others to respond. There are countless posts about suicide on this site. Although many of the responses are positive and hopeful, other responses are hurtful and dangerous, encouraging those who are suicidal to take their own lives. (It should be noted that recently, Whisper.sh has begun attempts to monitor these messages and remove harmful content.)

Practical strategy (parents): Once most adults have heard of dangerous Internet games or challenges, like the Blue Whale Game, it may well already be over. Therefore, although it's important to keep your eyes open and read the news to know what's trending, it's even more important to keep your ears open to listen to what's going on with your own child. As parents, you are already involved and passionate about so many aspects of your child's life—it's important not to let your child's online life be a mystery. We often hear parents say things like: "He's on the computer all the time. I don't know what he does—he's just a whiz! Whew, makes my head spin!" as though somehow because children are more nimble and advanced with computers and technology than their parents, they don't need adult supervision. Of course, that's not true. Talk to your child about what they are doing online and with whom they are doing it. And listen to what they tell you.

Now for the Good News: Technology, Social Media, and the Online World Might Be How to Fix This!

Of course, it is healthy to encourage children to spend time offline—to go for a walk, practice yoga, or just hang out with friends. However, that doesn't mean that online time is necessarily dangerous or bad. In fact, there is a growing body of research that suggests that online risks simply mirror offline vulnerabilities (see

Odgers & Jensen, 2020). These researchers argue that certain types of social media engagement may simply amplify existing mental health risks for certain adolescents. In other words, it may be that online risks are different for different youth, and those who are already at risk in the offline world continue to be at risk in the online world. They argue that the media hype about the negative effects of time spent on digital platforms has deflected attention away from the real problem, which is the heightened levels of mental health concerns among vulnerable youth.

The debate about the effects of time spent on digital devices will undoubtedly continue. Nevertheless, when it comes to suicide prevention, we know that if we are developing programming that only takes place offline, we are missing important opportunities to connect with students. We also are missing some very effective strategies to reach our students where they are and that engage them in exciting and interesting ways.

For every horror story about cyberbullying and suicide connected to social media, there are also countless stories of hope, caring, and lives saved. These stories, however, rarely make the news. Those of us who work in suicide prevention must constantly remind each other that we often know about the lives that are lost, but we seldom hear about the lives that are saved from the work that we do. The same is true for the positive effects of online communication.

Creating Connections: Being Confident, Competent, and Willing to Intervene

There are many ways that adolescents create connections in the virtual world. From the perspective of suicide prevention, the best virtual connections are with people who feel confident that they can assist, who are competent in giving them accurate information, and who are willing to be part of a positive intervention.

Connecting Online: More Than Just Finding Friends. Online communities can provide great support for people at risk for suicide, and there are many online sites that offer overall supportive atmospheres, either with caring moderators or with members, or both. Research finds that the majority of people who join Internet discussions about suicide, even those who initially join to find support for their suicide-related plans, ultimately have a reduction in suicide-related ideation after joining such a group, although this is not universally true. In some cases, suicide risk is heightened, and suicide is sometimes portrayed as a legitimate solution to problems (Robinson et al., 2016). Nevertheless, there is reason to believe that, *in general,* discussion groups can reduce suicide risk.

Social Media: When the Power of Networks Is Used for Good, Not for Evil. Social media can help suicidal adolescents. When young people post about their suicidal thoughts or plans on social media or other online venues, their posts are often met with care and concern, as well as practical advice, including links to the national hotline. Oftentimes, their peers reach out in person, or they tell parents, counselors, or others in the school, giving the adults a chance to intervene that would have been impossible without these online disclosures.

For youth who are isolated, either geographically or because they feel alone due to identities that differ from their classmates, social media also offers the opportunity to connect with others who share similar stories and offer connections that were unheard of just a few years ago. Marginalized youth, in particular, can benefit from the unique friendship groups and sources of support that specialized affinity networks can provide. For example, social media has opened up opportunities for LGBTQI+ youth to connect with one another and offer spaces of de-stigmatization and emotional support, and it is in these types of online communities that marginalized youth can begin to develop language and understanding of their own identity, to foster self-reflexivity, to practice self-disclosure, and to see role models for gender performativity (Ito et al., 2020). Importantly, these virtual connections are available at any time of the day or night, including times when marginalized youth may feel most vulnerable.

Clearly, social media offers an important type of connectivity, but there are many other positive venues for connection online. The mere act of having their content reblogged or reshared by others can make youth feel supported or valued (McCracken, 2017). Similarly, resharing the content of others is a way of showing support for them. Of course, we recognize the inherent dangers here of not having content sufficiently liked or shared. However, the importance of the decision to like or share makes the point that youth have many ways to feel supported online, and adults must be aware of the intensity of emotions that come with these seemingly simple acts. Fandom communities have been shown to increase the mental health of participants through many positive impacts, including increased connectedness, reduced isolation, reduced risky behaviors, and increased confidence and self-efficacy (Ito et al., 2019). Overall, when the virtual world works well, the sense of belonging that it offers to teens who crave the feeling of fitting in can be a powerful protective factor against suicide.

Just the Facts, Please.   The Internet also offers suicidal youth instant access to help and resources, and the digital world has a strong role to play in breaking down the stigma of help seeking. Today's students are much more accepting of mental illness and mental health care than previous generations. Nearly 90% of adolescents have gone online to seek out mental health– or suicide-related information or resources (Rideout & Fox, 2018). Simply type the word "suicide" into Google, and the first pages are all about help and resources. In other words, young people are seeking out information. Helping them locate and identify quality resources, and distinguish helpful and fact-based information from hype and hysteria, is one of the best suicide prevention skills students can learn.

Engaging in Digital Suicide Prevention

Many of the very aspects of the digital world that make it potentially dangerous for youth in the broader sense can actually be rather
helpful when it comes to suicide prevention. The relative anonymity
of online searching, the time of day (or night) when many students
use the Internet, and the fact that they often conduct their online
searches alone all might contribute to the likelihood that students will
use the Internet to gather important information about suicide prevention and mental health. In fact, we believe (and research will back
this up) that effective suicide prevention and intervention in the current age, particularly if it is geared toward children and adolescents,
absolutely must include digital components. Therefore, we encourage schools to integrate both face-to-face and digital formats in
all aspects of the prevention, intervention, and postvention strategies
that we discuss in the remaining chapters of this book.

In general, there are four major ways that schools can use digital
and electronic formats for suicide prevention with their students:

1. Schools can help students (and others) learn how to monitor
   the content of messages that they read online to notice and be
   aware of suicidal intent of others and, importantly, to know
   what to do.
2. Schools can use digital formats to help students (as well as
   teachers and staff) to learn suicide prevention strategies, such
   as suicide prevention education and gatekeeper training.
3. Schools can use digital media strategies as part of their suicide
   awareness and mental health advocacy campaigns.
4. Schools can teach students how to post appropriate positive
   content related to mental health and well-being, as well as suicide prevention resources, on Internet blogs and websites.

For each of these strategies, it is important and useful to involve and engage students in digital strategies to promote suicide

prevention. When adults create digital approaches on behalf of students, the strategies are less likely to be perceived as appropriate by the students or to be successful overall. Rather, including students, with appropriate adult supervision to monitor content, appears to be the most promising approach.

Practical strategy (schools): Whenever we interact with students about the digital world and suicide prevention, we remind them that they will be the generation that solves these problems, and we speak with them from a place of hope and optimism. We remember what it was like to have our parents tell us that the new technology or fads of our time (television, computers, rap music—whatever it was) would destroy civilization. Parents and others have issued these dire warnings to children for decades. It is true that there are reasons to be concerned about the overuse of technology in our children's lives. However, sending the message to our children that they cannot survive this, that it will destroy them, and that this is too much for them to handle will not help. Rather, we reassure them that they will use this very technology to manage these problems in ways that we, the older generation, do not understand and cannot even imagine. They are creative and enterprising. We will help. We will offer content and expertise. We will guide them, and we will make sure they are safe while they work to create solutions. Hope is essential to suicide prevention, and that includes hope about the digital world too. There are many reasons to be hopeful about the many good things that can happen online and the lives that can be saved with technology.

Conclusion

We know that the digital world, particularly social media, can seem overwhelming and frightening when it comes to suicide prevention.

There are, of course, countless horror stories of how students have been threatened, bullied, and cajoled into risky behaviors. Young people have learned how to escalate their suicidal thoughts or behaviors or even been pushed to suicide by their online involvement. Nevertheless, today's students live in an online environment. We must help them make sense of what they see, hear, and participate in when they engage in these virtual relationships so that they are protected and safe. We also believe that there is great potential in helping students use their engagement in these online platforms to help reduce mental health stigma, encourage help seeking, and lower suicidality. Although we don't have the answers, we also know that attempting to impose solutions on our students will not be met with much enthusiasm. Rather, school-based mental health professionals can teach appropriate guidelines and then support and encourage students as they discover how to best, and safely, use these virtual platforms.

References

American Foundation for Suicide Prevention. (2011). *Recommendations for reporting on suicide*. https://reportingonsuicide.org/

Bian, M. W., & Leung, L. (2015). Linking loneliness, shyness, smartphone addiction symptoms, and patterns of smartphone use to social capital. *Social Science Computer Review, 33*, 61–79. doi:10.1177/0894439314528779

Bridge, J. A., Greenhouse, J. B., Ruch, D., Stevens, J., Ackerman, J., Sheftall, A. H., Horowitz, L. M., Kelleher, K. J., & Campo, J. V. (2020). Association between the release of Netflix's 13 Reasons Why and suicide rates in the United States: An interrupted time series analysis. *Journal of the American Academy of Child & Adolescent Psychiatry, 59*(2), 236–243.

Butt, S., & Phillips, J. G. (2008). Personality and self reported mobile phone use. *Computers and Human Behavior, 24*, 346–360. doi:10.1016/j.chb.2007.01.019

Cohen-Almagor, R. (2018). Social responsibility on the Internet: Addressing the challenge of cyberbullying. *Aggression and Violent Behavior, 39*, 42–52.

Common Sense Media. (2019). *Media use by tweens and teens 2019: Infographic*. https://commonsensemedia.org/Media-use-by-tweens-and-teens-2019-infographic

Dagar, A., & Falcone, T. (2020). High viewership of videos about teen suicide on YouTube. *Journal of the American Academic of Child and Adolescent Psychiatry, 59*(1), 1–3.

Desk, E. W. (2017, September 6). *What is the Blue Whale Challenge?* http://indianexpress.com/article/whatis/what-is-the-blue-whale-challenge/

Granello, D. H. (1997). Using "Beverly Hills 90210" to explore developmental issues in female adolescents [A qualitative analysis]. *Youth and Society, 29,* 24–53.

Hackett, L. (2020). *Ditch the label.* https://www.ditchthelabel.org

Hakoyama, M. (2019). Young adults' cellphone dependence, stress, depression and self-esteem. *Advances in Social Science and Culture, 1*(2), 125–142.

Hinduja, S., & Patchin, J. W. (2018a). *What to do when your child is cyberbullied: Top ten tips for parents.* Cyberbullying Research Center. https://cyberbullying.org/tips-for-parents-when-your-child-is-cyberbullied.pdf

Hinduja, S., & Patchin, J. W. (2018b). *Preventing cyberbullying: Top ten tips for educators.* Cyberbullying Research Center. https://cyberbullying.org/Top-Ten-Tips-Educators-Cyberbullying-Prevention.pdf

Ito, M., Baumer, S., Bittanti, M., Boyd, D., Cody, R., Stephenson, B. H., Horst, H. A., Lange, P. G., Mahendran, D., Martínez, K. Z., Pascoe, C. J., Perkel, D., Robinson, L., Sims, C., & Tripp, L. (2019). *Hanging out, messing around, and geeking out: Kids living and learning with new media* (10th anniversary ed.). MIT Press.

Ito, M., Odgers, C., Schueller, S., Cabrera, J., Conaway, E., Cross, R., & Hernandez, M. (2020). *Social media and youth wellbeing: What we know and where we could go.* Connected Learning Alliance.

Jaitly, T., Nair, S., Gupta, S., & Shukla, S. K. (2018). Manipulative suicides: A new paradigm of suggestive deaths among adolescents and young adults. *Research Journal of Humanities and Social Sciences, 9*(3), 529–534.

Joiner, T. E. (2005). *Why people die by suicide.* Harvard University Press.

Katapally, T. R., Laxer, R., Qian, W., & Leatherdale, S. T. (2017). Do school physical activity policies and programs have a role in decreasing multiple screen time behaviours among youth? *Preventative Medicine, 110,* 106–111. doi:10.1016/j.ypmed.2017.11.026

Kim, D. J., Kim, J. Y., & Pyeon, A. P. M. (2016). Altered functional connectivity related smartphone overuse in adolescent. *International Journal of Neuropsychopharmacology, 19*(9), 9. doi:1093/ijnp/pyw041.306

Kim, M-H., Min, S., Ahn, J-S., An, C., & Lee, J. (2019). Association between high adolescent smartphone use and academic impairment, conflicts with family members or friends, and suicide attempts. *PLoS ONE, 14*(7), e0219831. doi:10.1371/journal.pone.0219831

Kowalski, R., Limber, S., & Agatston, P. W. (2008). *Cyber bullying.* Blackwell.

Luxton, D. D., June, J. D., & Fairall, J. M. (2012). Social media and suicide: A public health perspective, *American Journal of Public Health, 102*(S2), S195–S200. doi:10.2105/AJPH.2011.300608

McCracken, A. (2017). Tumblr youth subcultures and media engagement. *Cinema Journal, 57*(1), 151–161.

Nuccitelli, M. (2020). *42 Examples of cyberbullying & cyberbullying tactics.* https://www.ipredator.co/examples-of-cyberbullying

Odgers, C. L., & Jensen, J. R. (2020). Annual research review: Adolescent mental health in the digital age: Facts, fears, and future directions. *Journal of Child Psychology and Psychiatry, 61*(3), 336–348.

Patchin, J. W. (2018). *More on the link between bullying and suicide.* Cyberbullying Research Center. https://cyberbullying.org/more-on-the-link-between-bullying-and-suicide

Pew Research Center. (2018a). *Teens, social media & technology 2018.* https://www.pewresearch.org/internet/2018/05/31/teens-social-media-technology-2018/

Pew Research Center. (2018b). *A majority of teens have experienced some form of cyberbullying.* https://www.pewresearch.org/internet/2018/09/27/a-majority-of-teens-have-experienced-some-form-of-cyberbullying/pi_2018-09-27_teens-and-cyberbullying_0-01/

Rideout, V., & Fox, S. (2018). *Digital health practices, social media use, and mental well-being among teens in the U.S.* Hopelab/Well-being Trust. https://hopelab.org/reports/pdf/a-national-survey-by-hopelab-and-well-being-trust-2018.pdf

Robinson, J., Cox, G., Bailey, E., Hetrick, S., Rodrigues, M., Fisher, S., & Herrman, H. (2016). Social media and suicide prevention: A systematic review. *Early Intervention in Psychiatry, 10*, 103–121.

Statista.com. (2020). *Percentage of teenagers in the United States who have access to a desktop or laptop computer at home as of April 2018, by age group.* https://www.statista.com/statistics/475949/usage-of-desktop-latop-teens-age/

Twenge, J. M., Joiner, T. E., Rogers, M. L., & Martin, G. H. (2017). Increases in depressive symptoms, suicide-related outcomes, and suicide rates among U.S. adolescents after 2010 and links to increased new media screen time. *Clinical Psychological Science, 6*(1), 3–17. doi:10.1177/2167702617723376

5

Self-Injury

Understanding Students Who Engage in Self-Harm

As we move to this chapter about self-injury, which is a bit of a departure from the previous chapters, we'd like to start with a story. As you read through it, we encourage you to pay attention not only to what you think you would do if you encountered this student but also to your emotional reactions to both the student and the situation.

Sarah is a 13-year-old girl and a middle schooler. She is quiet, has average grades, and has never caused any problems. At the moment, she lives with her grandmother because her mother is in a residential treatment center for substance dependency. Her parents are divorced, and Sarah hasn't seen her father since she was in the first grade. Recently, one of her teachers saw Sarah in the lunchroom, pulling up her sweatshirt sleeves to show her forearms to another girl in her class. The teacher saw that Sarah's arms were filled with numerous cuts, many of which appeared to be recently inflicted. Concerned, the teacher sent Sarah to the school nurse, who bandaged the cuts and talked briefly with Sarah. Sarah refused to answer directly when the school nurse asked if she is currently suicidal. She said she has thought about suicide in the past and thought "when the time came," she would probably die by cutting herself too deep. In the meantime, she said she needs to cut in order to feel better. "It takes my mind off everything that builds up inside of me."

Suicide and Self-Injury in Schools. Darcy Haag Granello, Paul F. Granello, Gerald A. Juhnke,
Oxford University Press. © Oxford University Press 2023. DOI: 10.1093/oso/9780190059842.003.0005

In our work with teachers, counselors, school psychologists, administrators, and other school mental health professionals throughout the United States, we are increasingly confronted with stories like Sarah's. If you were speaking with Sarah, we're sure you'd have a lot of questions for her in order to better understand what is causing her to self-injure. You might wonder how long Sarah has been cutting or if she engages in any other types of self-injury. You might have questions about any other unhealthy coping strategies she might use, such as substances or isolating or withdrawing from others. You might also wonder if she is depressed or anxious, or because self-injury is a symptom of borderline personality disorder, you might even wonder if she is on her way to developing a personality disorder. And if you are like the school nurse in the story, you probably wonder if Sarah's self-injurious behaviors are connected to thoughts of suicide.

In this chapter, we will give you information about nonsuicidal self-injury (NSSI) among K–12 students, an increasingly common behavior that causes deep levels of concern among school mental health personnel, parents, and even many young people themselves. NSSI is a complex behavior with biological, psychological, and social variables that make understanding NSSI extraordinarily challenging. Adding to the complexity are the strong negative emotional reactions that many people have to youth who self-injure that make working with these students particularly difficult. Teachers and school mental health professionals tell us that they simply want more information and practical guidelines to help them work with students who engage in NSSI behaviors, and we understand the desire for clear answers and the comfort that comes with best practice guidelines. Although a comprehensive text on clinical and intervention strategies is beyond the scope of this book, we will give you the most up-to-date information and point you to resources to help you work with students who have already been identified as engaging in NSSI. In short, we will do our best to offer what research supports.

What might be most compelling about NSSI, at least for the purpose of this book, is the question of whether, or how, NSSI is connected to suicide risk in children and adolescents. In our work presenting suicide trainings around the country and internationally, we are increasingly being asked about the relationship of NSSI behavior to suicide. Because this is a book about suicide and suicide prevention, understanding this link and developing prevention strategies for NSSI will be the focal point of our chapter. It's an important conversation, which is why we have dedicated a chapter specifically to this topic. Before we move to that discussion, let's start by understanding just what we mean by NSSI, how many students are involved, and who is most likely to engage in self-injury.

NSSI: Children Who Hurt Themselves

NSSI, sometimes called deliberate self-harm, is the intentional, self-inflicted destruction of body tissue that results in immediate damage, without intent to die and for purposes that are not culturally sanctioned. Although there are many different types of injury, the most common are as follows:

- Carving or cutting into the skin
- Burning oneself
- Punching or hitting oneself or throwing oneself down the stairs
- Headbanging
- Embedding objects under the skin

Although self-injury can occur anywhere on the body, it most often occurs on the hands, wrists, arms, stomach, and thighs. The severity of self-injury can range from very superficial scratches to injuries that permanently disfigure or cause life-threatening wounds. In general, tattoos or body piercing are not considered

NSSI unless they are done for the sole purpose of harming the body (Muehlenkamp et al., 2018).

Understanding Who Is at Risk

In schools across the country, about one in five students (18% in high schools, about 20% in middle schools) has engaged in NSSI at least once over the past year. At least some of these students, perhaps as many as half, engage in severe, chronic self-injury. Certainly for the majority of those who engage in self-injury, it is not a single behavior. Rather, it is something that lasts for weeks, months, or even years. For most people, self-injury is a behavior that is cyclical rather than linear. That is, it starts, continues for a period of time, stops, and then resumes.

The Rates of NSSI Are on the Rise: Is This More Cases or Higher Levels of Reporting?

It's hard to know whether the higher rates of NSSI come from an actual increase in the number of students who are engaging in self-harm or simply a growing awareness of the problem. What is clear is that the number of NSSI cases being identified in schools is growing. In the last several decades, there has been a sharp increase in the level of social consciousness of NSSI. There have been more and more portrayals of self-harm on television, in movies, and on the Internet and an exponential growth of NSSI-focused research and media stories. Further, there are now thousands of websites on the topic, videos on YouTube, and Instagram pictures that portray NSSI behavior to youth. Popular youth icons, such as Megan Fox, Johnny Depp, Miley Cyrus, Demi Lovato, and Angelina Jolie, have all publicly discussed their struggles with self-injuring behaviors. In fact, there is so much attention paid to NSSI in the media that as of 2020, there are media guidelines for the responsible reporting and depicting of NSSI (Westers et al., 2021).

This increase in awareness among both the adolescent population and school-based professionals has led to the identification of more cases, even if the actual rate of these cases in the population is not increasing. Nevertheless, whether the actual rate of NSSI is increasing or not probably doesn't matter, since the reality is that more and more youth with NSSI behavior are identified in schools, and schools must respond appropriately.

The Severity of NSSI Varies Greatly

Self-injury occurs on a spectrum—from superficial scratches to life-threatening injuries that can permanently disable or disfigure. In general, NSSI methods such as superficial cutting, scratching, punching, and burning are not life-threatening. Nevertheless, NSSI behaviors certainly can cross the line and become quite life-threatening, even unintentionally. We worked with a young woman who intended to cut herself on the arm to help ameliorate emotional pain but ended up with deep lacerations that bled so much that she required a lengthy hospital stay and skin grafts to repair the damage. The nerves in her arm were lacerated, and she never recovered full function or feeling in her hand or arm. The damage was permanent. Her case mirrors the nearly 20% of adolescents who say that their NSSI behaviors got out of control, and they ended up hurting themselves more seriously than they intended (Whitlock, 2018). The point is, although lethality is often rather low with NSSI, permanent damage, or death, can and does occur.

Practical strategy (schools): Although self-injury is relatively common, it often goes undetected. All school personnel should have basic awareness of signs that a student may be engaging in self-harm and be trained to know what to do when they suspect someone is at risk for NSSI. Arms, fists, and forearms opposite the dominant hands are a common place for injury (particularly among girls), although evidence can occur anywhere on the body. Other signs include the following:

- *Inappropriate dress for the season (especially consistently wearing long sleeves or long pants in warm weather)*
- *Consistent use of wrist bands or other wrist coverings*
- *Unexplained scars or bruising*
- *Unwillingness to participate in events or activities that require less body coverage (such as swimming/gym class), even if culturally appropriate*
- *Secretive behaviors (e.g., lots of time in the bathroom or other isolated areas)*
- *Frequent bandages*
- *Odd or unexplainable objects in lockers or on their person (e.g., razor blades, implements that could be used to cut or pound)*
- *Increased isolation or withdrawal*
- *Increased depression, anxiety, or other strong negative emotions, such as anger, rage, fear, or self-loathing*

It Is Commonly Believed That More Girls Than Boys Engage in NSSI. This Is Uncertain. For years, it was assumed that females are at higher risk for NSSI than males. Surveys consistently find that girls report higher rates of NSSI than boys, with the gap between girls and boys growing wider as children move from elementary through middle and into high school. In high school, nearly 3 times as many girls as boys report that they engage in NSSI. Overall, among all students, girls are more than twice as likely to report that they engage in repetitive self-injury (rNSSI). This is consistent with the higher rates of self-reported depression, eating disorders, anxiety, and other emotional disorders among girls. Recently, however, at least some scholars have begun to question whether these self-reported rates are accurate and whether there are true differences in rates of self-injury between the sexes.

Regardless of rates, there clearly are gendered differences in *how* students engage in NSSI. In general, among middle and high school students, girls report more scratching and cutting and are more likely to injure themselves in the arms and legs. Boys are more likely to engage in burning and hitting-type behavior and more likely to injure themselves in the chest, face, or genitals (Sornberger et al., 2012).

Unlike boys, girls are more likely to engage in self-injury alone. However, once they have engaged in the self-injury, girls are more likely to share their scars or their stories as a way of seeking attention, solace or care, or belonging. Once hurt, girls also are more likely to seek medical attention for their self-injury (Whitlock, 2018).

When adolescent boys engage in self-injury, it appears that their methods, and their reasons, differ from the ways in which girls engage in these behaviors. However, because for years it was assumed that boys simply did not engage in self-injury at very high rates, the research and understanding of NSSI among boys lag that of girls. Therefore, it is more difficult for us to make clear statements about NSSI among boys. Here is the current state of research and clinical work.

Boys, particularly those who believe they should follow more hypermasculine ways of being, are more likely to wound themselves more severely. They are also less likely than girls to seek appropriate medical care for wounds. They are more likely to engage in injuries that involve punching themselves, throwing themselves into objects or walls, or dropping heavy objects on their bodies. Adolescent boys are much more likely to engage in self-injury with other boys, and some may engage in NSSI with a peer group (e.g., "blood brothers") or in response to a dare from peers (Green & Jakupak, 2016). Whereas girls typically seek social support, attention, or solace from their self-injury, adolescent boys who self-injure in this way may derive positive reinforcement in the form of social status among the peer group and approval from others for their NSSI (e.g., being "tough" or "badass"). For others, self-harm can be used as a method to communicate to others that they should not be "messed with" and should be left alone. Finally, at least for some adolescent boys, self-injury is a form of self-punishment or a strategy to handle frustration (Whitlock, 2018).

All of these differences in how adolescents engage in NSSI might help explain the differences in survey responses. For adolescent boys who incorporate NSSI into their vision of masculinity, it may be unrealistic to assume they will admit to self-harm on school surveys. Certainly, for at least some of these boys following a hypermasculine script, there would be little incentive to "report" these self-harm behaviors to perceived "authorities." Additionally, the type of self-injury preferred by adolescent boys (bruising in hidden places) can either go undetected by others or be viewed as less serious as the cutting in visible places that is often the preferred method of adolescent girls. Finally, because girls are more likely to seek help for their self-injury and their injuries are more likely to align with public perceptions of self-injury, it may simply be that there is a lack of awareness among school personnel about self-injury among boys. For these reasons, self-injury among boys can be left out of school reports or minimized by those who engage in it. Nevertheless, national data sets consistently find that nearly a quarter of females aged 14–18 say they have engaged in NSSI during that previous year, compared with approximately 14% of males (Centers for Disease Control and Prevention [CDC], 2019).

Practical strategy (schools): It is clear that all school personnel need training and education in NSSI. Teachers and staff may end up being "first responders." Wester et al. (2017) recommend that, at the very least, all staff should receive in-service training about NSSI, what it is, how to identify it, how to respond to a student who engages in or talks about NSSI, how to have conversations about effective and healthy coping strategies, and personnel students can reach out to for help within the school. We would add that the in-service training should include discussion about gendered differences in self-harm to ensure that school personnel recognize implicit gendered assumptions they might be making about self-harm and to help them recognize and reach out to boys who may be at risk.

Younger Students Engage in NSSI at Higher Rates . Those with early-onset NSSI can engage in these behaviors as early as 7 years old, but most students begin this behavior around ages 12–14. The overall pattern is that middle schoolers have higher rates than high school students, with a slow and steady decline in rates as students age. For many students who engage in NSSI, it appears that these behaviors tend to subside after about 5 years, although for others, the behaviors continue, at least into early adulthood. What differentiates these two groups, those who stop the behaviors during adolescence and those who persist beyond high school, is unclear.

Practical strategy (schools): We are often asked when is "too early" to have classroom guidance specifically about suicide prevention or self-injury. Our standard answer is that we need to begin laying the groundwork with elementary-aged children. The research is clear that it is essential to teach children healthy coping, including emotional regulation, help seeking, loneliness prevention, and effective problem-solving, which are all strategies that help prevent the onset of unhealthy coping in later years. Primary prevention efforts at the elementary level that include emotion identification may be particularly helpful given the relationship between NSSI and the inability to correctly identify and label emotions (Cerutti et al., 2014).

Latinx Students Have Elevated Risk, but Students of Every Race and Ethnicity Are at Risk.   It is difficult to fully understand the role that race and ethnicity play in risk for NSSI. Traditionally, NSSI was seen as primarily a concern for White females, but recent data calls this into question. What is now clear is that NSSI is a problem among students of all races and ethnicities. However, it appears that Latinx youth self-injure at significantly higher rates: 26% of middle school students, which is significantly higher than either White (19%) or Black (16%) students, and 30% of high school students, which is much higher than either White (17%) or Black (17%) students (CDC, 2019). The take-home message is certainly that NSSI can no longer be considered a problem that exists only, or indeed even primarily, among White females. This is a problem that transcends race, ethnicity, and sex.

LGBTQI+Students Engage in NSSI at Higher Rates. Students who identify as LGBTQI+ engage in NSSI at higher rates than their heterosexual or cisgender peers, with rates that may be up to 3 times higher (DeCamp & Bakken, 2016). Research is limited, but it is probable that higher rates of depression, peer victimization, and substance abuse, as well as health-related risk behaviors, such as disordered eating, contribute to these elevated rates. There is some (mixed) evidence that, at least for some adolescent boys who identify as attracted to other boys, engaging in same-sex sexual activity is correlated with increased rates of NSSI (DeCamp & Bakken, 2016). This reminds us that the adolescent world is extremely complicated—perhaps even more so for LGBTQI+ youth. Of course, correlation is *not causation*, and engaging in same-sex sexual activity does not cause NSSI. It appears, however, that *at least for some youth*, engaging in sexual activity is fraught with emotions that may be difficult to process and could potentially contribute to NSSI behaviors (although this is certainly not true for all of the boys in all of the studies). In general, however, these findings underscore the importance of positive role models for all students in the school, and in particular, for youth who identify as gay and bisexual.

Practical strategy (schools): Improving school culture for LGBTQI+ youth, including providing support groups, has been shown to reduce victimization, suicide attempts, and NSSI (NYC Health,

2017). In addition, providing positive role models, particularly gay males, who are willing to speak about positive methods for coping is one very specific strategy that schools can use to help limit NSSI behaviors among their students who identify as LGBTQI+.

Many Risk Factors Contribute to NSSI, With Similar Risks That Contribute to Suicide Risk. It is perhaps not surprising that many of the same factors that place children and adolescents at risk for suicide also contribute to their risk for NSSI. Among those that are best understood are history of trauma, abuse, or neglect; difficulty with emotional regulation; presence of other mental health conditions, most often depression, anxiety, and disordered eating; low self-compassion; and exposure to NSSI (Wester et al., 2017).

Practical strategy (schools): Although intervention efforts specifically designed to address the risk factors associated with NSSI are important, programs that help address any of the mental health conditions that are associated with NSSI and teach students positive coping strategies can have the effects of lowering NSSI behaviors among the student population.

Understanding Why Students Engage in NSSI

Now that you have a sense of what NSSI is and which and how many students are likely to engage in it, let's turn to the more difficult question of *why* students might engage self-harm. As we move to this discussion, we are also painfully aware that a significant proportion of readers of this book have *their own stories* of self-harm. If you have your own history of (or are currently engaging in) self-harm, we encourage you to engage in self-care. This is difficult material for all of us—particularly for those with their own histories and stories. As always, this isn't just about our students—it is also about ourselves. Please take care of yourself. Get the help you need, and be ever mindful that these discussions can be difficult and triggering.

Practical strategy (self): If you find yourself triggered by the information in this chapter (or in this book), we encourage you to stop reading and seek professional help. This is also true for working with students who self-harm. The work that we do is important and rewarding, but it can also feel depleting and exhausting. If you have had your own experiences with self-harm, your empathy for students who are hurting themselves can be a powerful motivator to keep you engaged—perhaps more than you would with other students. Your own experiences with self-harm clearly bring you a level of understanding and compassion that others may not have, and that can be rewarding—but it can draw you in deeper. Your involvement with these students can even trigger your own cycle of self-injury. When your involvement leads to your own thoughts of self-harm, then you have crossed over an important line. Remember, an important message we tell our students when we teach them to help others is "get help for yourself first." That holds for us too.

There Are Many Reasons Why People Engage in NSSI

The "why" of self-injury is complex. We believe that for most people, there are biological, psychological, and social variables that combine to make the individual adopt the behavior. To complicate NSSI even further, a single act of self-injury can serve multiple purposes, and the reasons that a person engages in NSSI can change over time.

Although it can be challenging to understand the complexity of NSSI behaviors, it may be useful to think of the motivators behind the behaviors using a model composed of four components (You et al., 2018): (a) automatic-negative reinforcement (A-NR),

(b) automatic-positive reinforcement (A-PR), (c) social-positive reinforcement (S-PR), and (d) social-negative reinforcement (S-NR). In this model, automatic simply means internal, existing within the youth. From this perspective, then, those who engage in NSSI do so essentially because of internally derived negative (A-NR) or positive (A-PR) emotional states or from externally derived (social) positive (S-PR) or negative (S-NR) motivations. We can think of the NSSI behaviors as the youth's attempts to get rid of negative emotions (A-NR), to feel positive emotions (A-PR), to communicate something to others (S-PR), or to escape external demands or control the reactions of others (S-NR). The words the students use can often tip us off to the motivations behind their behaviors. For example, when we hear words like "I feel out of control" or "I am overwhelmed by sadness," we understand that the student is motivated by their negative emotions (A-NR). When students say, "I just wanted to feel something" or "I needed to feel real," we understand that this comes from a place of needing to feel positive emotions (A-NR). Other motivations come from the student's interactions with others. For example, "I want you to know how I am feeling" or "I want my counselor to . . ." are signals that the self-harm is being used to demonstrate the intensity of their feelings to the outside world (S-PR). Finally, "I do it to get people to back off and leave me alone" or "I wanted to freak out my mom" are clear examples of controlling others (S-NR).

We know this is a lot, so we'll discuss these four basic motivations in more detail below. We want to take some time with this model because understanding what is behind an individual's NSSI behaviors will ultimately help guide the therapeutic interventions for a particular student. In other words, once we understand what the young person is trying to accomplish with the NSSI behaviors, we have a better chance to intervene.

It's important to note that in most schools, outside providers will work with students to provide these intense intervention strategies, and this type of therapeutic intervention is typically not within the job duties of the school counselor, school psychologist, school social worker, or school nurse. In all cases, the mental health professionals within the school building should follow their professional standards of care, ethics, and expectations of the school administration when providing care to their students and should have a clear understanding of their professional boundaries. In most cases, that means they will not be providing this type of therapeutic intervention. Nevertheless, we believe it is still useful to have a conceptual model to understand NSSI behaviors, even if students are receiving their mental health care from external providers. It is helpful that school personnel and external providers are on the same page. Finally, as we move on, we note that although each of these four components of the model provides a meaningful perspective for understanding NSSI, for adolescents the most common reason given for NSSI is to cope with intense negative feelings. For that reason, that is where we will begin.

Most Students Who Engage in Self-Harm Say It Is for Emotional Regulation. Although there are many reasons that young people say they hurt themselves, the majority say they do it because they are experiencing intense negative emotions that they cannot fully understand and cannot process. They self-injure to manage that pain or to cope with the intensity of their feelings. Some say that if they have physical pain, they can focus on that pain instead of their intense emotional pain. These students sometimes say that when the knife was removed or the hitting stopped, they felt what it was like to *not* to be in pain, which felt like a relief. These students fall into the A-NR component of the model. These students have intense negative emotions that they have never learned to fully identify, understand, or express. They turn to self-injury to help them process these negative emotions.

Some of the most common negative emotions associated with self-injury are self-hatred, shame, guilt, and anger, although any negative emotions can contribute to the desire to self-harm if the student has not learned to regulate them. Students might speak of self-loathing and the need to punish themselves. Others may discuss a pattern of stress, pressure, frustration, or anger building up to intolerable levels, and self-injury as a strategy for release. This cycle is familiar to anyone who works in mental health. We see this same cycle in many impulse control disorders, as well as cycles of abuse, violence, and addiction. There is a period of building tension that leads to an incident, often followed by guilt or remorse, a period of calm, and, ultimately, rising tension again. For some, rather than a period of calm, the guilt and remorse over the incident become part of the negative emotion that feeds the cycle. And the pattern continues. To break the cycle, we must give young people alternate ways of managing and processing their negative emotions before they escalate to the point where they see no other alternative but to use pain to process them.

Practical strategy (schools): Adolescents who engage in NSSI often share six key problems with emotional dysregulation: (a) lack of awareness of emotional responses, (b) lack of clarity of emotional responses, (c) nonacceptance of emotional responses, (d) limited access to emotional regulation strategies that they perceive as effective, (e) difficulties controlling impulses when experiencing negative emotions, and (f) difficulties engaging in goal-directed behaviors when experiencing negative emotions (Gratz & Romer, 2004). Helping students learn strategies to address any of these core elements could play an important role in reducing NSSI behaviors.

Some People Self-Injure in Order to Feel Something. A second internally derived motivation for NSSI is the desire to *feel something—anything.* Students who self-injure for this reason often say that they feel emotionally numb and that the physical pain of the self-harm allows them to feel *something.* They may speak of a rush of energy (11%) or a good feeling that surges over their body (16%; Whitlock, 2018). Remember, emotional numbing can be part of depression, and the desire to feel again can be powerful—some even call it "addicting." Some of these students say that the physical pain allows them to cry, and that is the emotional release they need. These students might also say that they are using NSSI to distract themselves. When you hear students use words that sound like "emptiness," "numbing," or "nothingness," then you are encountering NSSI derived from A-PR.

Some People Use Self-Injury as a Way to Fit In or to Communicate to Others.   smaller percentage of youth who engage in NSSI state that they do so because they hope that someone will notice (about 18%) or even because they are doing it as part of a group who have all agreed to engage in self-harm (2%–3%; Whitlock, 2018). These students are engaging in self-injury derived from an S-PR perspective. Clearly, being motivated to self-injure by social needs differs from being motivated primarily from internal needs, but it is also clear that students can have multiple reasons for engaging in self-harm. Nevertheless, regardless of the initial motivation for the self-harm, the consequences—even if unintended—can be reinforcing. In other words, although students may not have originally engaged in NSSI to seek attention from (or even to shock) someone else, these reactions can become reinforcing and can contribute to the likelihood of future events. Therefore, parents and school personnel must be trained to have appropriate responses that do not increase the potential for future self-harm.

Practical strategy (parents): Although it can be frightening to learn that a child is engaging in self-injury and it may be tempting to deny the problem, yell, or even threaten or punish a child who is engaging in NSSI, the best thing to do is to take a deep breath, calm down, and listen. Remember that at least part of the motivation for the self-injury may be to see the reactions of others. A calm, caring, and nonjudgmental response is best. Reassure your child that you care and want to get them help from a mental health professional. Create an open dialogue and let them know you want to listen. Use statements that promote a desire to understand (e.g., "I know you might not even know why you do this. It's OK. We can talk about it"). Avoid statements that are blaming or demand that your child simply stop the behavior, which they may be unable to do on their own (e.g., "You'll have to wear long sleeves so no one sees those scars" or "You said you don't want to keep hurting yourself, so I don't know why you don't just stop").

*Practical strategy (schools): School personnel should follow a similar approach as parents, using calm, caring, and nonjudgmental language. There are two extremes that teachers and other school staff sometimes take, and **neither is helpful**. Sometimes, school staff show excessive interest in students who self-injure. Thinking they are being helpful, they talk to the student about their self-harm, encouraging the student to discuss details and show scars and bruises, and even permit the student to "relive" the moment when the self-harm occurred. These adults believe they are being supportive by listening to, and encouraging the telling of, the stories. However, this type of attention can actually reinforce the secondary gain of attention and encourage future self-harm. The second reaction that some school staff might have is to avert their eyes from the student—to be so concerned that they might unintentionally place their gaze on the student's wounds or bruises that they refuse to look at the student at all. These adults also think they are being supportive by giving the student "privacy" or not "embarrassing" them. However, this lack of attention can inadvertently prevent the student from talking to adults or seeking assistance in the future. Instead, statements that are delivered in a calm, dispassionate tone are best (e.g., "I have noticed that you have some cuts that appear to be fresh, and maybe self-inflicted. Would you be willing to tell me more about those?" or "I know it can be scary to talk about this stuff or to ask for help, but I believe that there are people who can help you"). Statements that threaten or escalate are not helpful (e.g., "If you don't stop cutting yourself, I'm going to have to tell your parents"). For more tips and suggestions, see https://www.self-injury.org.au/.*

Still Others Use Self-Injury to Push People Away. The fourth major category that explains the motivation for student self-injury is to keep others at a distance. Some youth say they are trying to shock or hurt someone else (about 6%). As we discussed earlier, boys in particular might use their self-injury to prove to others that they are "tough" and should be left alone. But both boys and girls can engage in NSSI to distance themselves from others—to further isolate and withdraw. We worked with one young woman whose parents were wealthy and successful. When she showed us her scars, she said, "This will prove to my dad that all the money in the world can't buy him a beautiful daughter." Although she had other reasons for hurting herself (depression, anxiety, and other mental health concerns), at least part of her rationale was that her NSSI would hurt someone else. This is the S-NR component of the model.

Self-Injury Can Help Some People Feel Better: There is one other major reason that people self-injure, and it doesn't fit neatly into the model we have been discussing. Emerging research is helping us to form a better picture, and it is becoming clearer that in addition to the four behavioral patterns described above, people also engage in self-harm as a way to feel better physically. It may sound counterintuitive, and the biological reasons are a bit complicated and beyond the scope of this text (see Störkel et al., 2021 for details on this emerging field of research). Nevertheless, in very simple terms, there are two main takeaways. First, it seems that people who self-injure process both emotional and physical reactions differently than those who do not. Second, because of the overlap in the way the brain processes emotional and physical pain, changes in physical pain can result in changes to emotional pain. This creates a powerful incentive for people to process emotional pain through changes to physical pain.

Okay, that's a lot of information, so let's take these one at a time. First, there are differences in the way that people who self-injure process pain. In general, research shows that those who engage in self-injury have higher reactivity to emotional stimuli.

They are more likely to have strong emotional reactions to ordinary situations. In other words, when two students experience the same thing, one student may simply be *biologically wired* to have a stronger emotional reaction. We don't know why. It may be because of early childhood experiences, trauma, coexisting mental health diagnoses, adverse childhood experience scores, environmental factors, or other reasons. What we do know is that for some children and adolescents, when faced with an external stimulus, their emotional reactions will be stronger. In addition, once these students have more extreme emotional reactions, they will have difficulty regulating their reactions. People who engage in self-injury tend to have difficulty with de-escalation. They do not know how to self-soothe, or how to "down-regulate" negative emotions, regardless of the source of their arousal. Finally, once these students are emotionally aroused, it appears that their perceptions of physical pain become lowered. We find this fascinating. In other words, there is a difference between young people who self-injure and those who do not in how they rate their perception of physical pain when they are emotionally aroused. Students who have engaged in NSSI have a higher pain threshold and do not rate physical pain as high as students who have not engaged in NSSI behaviors (Whitlock, 2018). The implications are clear. If these students do not feel as much physical pain, then there is less reason for them to be fearful of harming themselves. And when they do hurt themselves, they are more likely to do real damage.

The second biological process at play is the way the brain processes emotional and physical pain in all of us—not just those who self-injure. Our brains have overlap in how we process physical and emotional pain, meaning that if we decrease our physical pain, we can have the sensation that our emotional pain is also decreasing. Although there are different neural pathways in the brain for physical and emotional pain, a landmark study in 2013 proved that the interconnected nature of the brain means that the effects on our brain are virtually the same for both types of pain

(Meerwijk et al., 2013). In other words, if we increase, or decrease, our physical arousal, we simultaneously increase, or decrease, our emotional arousal. We know this, of course. This is why relaxation strategies work or why we tell ourselves to take a deep breath when we feel stressed or anxious. We inherently know that if we lower our physical arousal, it will help with our emotional arousal. Unfortunately, for those who self-injure, this link between physical and emotional pain has an unintentional effect. It means that if they hurt themselves physically, *when the physical pain subsides, the emotional hurt lessens too.* Therefore, when they are seeking to reduce their emotional pain, elevating their physical pain until it matches the emotional pain and then bringing both types of pain down together can be an effective strategy. It is for this reason that we need to help those who engage in NSSI find other ways to raise and lower their physical arousal as a strategy to manipulate their emotional arousal, too.

Practical strategy (schools): The powerful link between physical and emotional pain can be dangerous. It can also be a useful way to help students learn to engage in emotional de-escalation through physical de-escalation. For example, autogenics is a relaxation technique that teaches participants to control certain physiological variables (such as body temperature or blood pressure) through meditation or guided imagery. Simple autogenic phrases, focused on heaviness and warmth (e.g., "My arms are very heavy" and "My hands are warm"), repeated over and over, have been found to be effective in changing the body's physical state, ultimately reducing tension and anxiety.

Prevention of NSSI Behavior in Schools

At a minimum, school mental health professionals who want to lower the incidence of NSSI behaviors in their schools should do three things: (a) reduce communication about NSSI in the school and among peer groups, (b) reduce any public displays of scars and wounds, and (c) provide short-term psychoeducational counseling to individual students who are at risk (Walsh, 2006). However, there is certainly room for a much more proactive approach, one outlined by Wester et al. (2017), and one that we recommend as well. We believe that school mental health professionals should take a leadership role in helping students to learn emotional regulation and coping skills to help prevent the onset of self-harming behaviors. These emotional regulation skills are most often taught though developmentally appropriate classroom guidance lessons.

It is important to note that we *do not recommend* classroom guidance lessons or, indeed, any workshops or trainings directly involving students on NSSI itself. That is because we do not yet have sufficient evidence that these types of trainings are safe for all students. It is possible that education and training that discusses NSSI directly could inadvertently be triggering and could lead to an increase in behaviors. We want to note that there is one program that is available, called Signs of Self-Injury (SOSI; Muehlenkamp et al., 2010). SOSI is a universal education approach for reducing self-injury in high schools. It is similar to the universal suicide prevention program Signs of Suicide (SOS), and uses a similar premise. SOSI is designed to increase knowledge of NSSI behaviors, including warning signs and risk factors; to improve attitudes for help seeking; to lower stigma; and to increase help-seeking behaviors among youth who engage in NSSI. There are modules for staff and faculty. In addition, a student module uses video vignettes to teach students how to reach out to others. Although the initial research on SOSI was promising, there has been very little research on its effectiveness since the 2010 study. Clearly, more research is needed, and the SOSI program is not yet considered a "best practice" model. At present, it is the only universal education approach available for schools that has any empirical support. Nevertheless, we believe that we are on much firmer ground when we say that all training and education that involves students should be about healthy coping, processing negative emotions, and strategies to lower emotional arousal.

> *Practical strategy (schools): Classroom guidance strategies that teach students how to appropriately identify, label, and regulate emotions are essential. It is worth noting that youth who engage in NSSI behaviors are more likely to use a higher number of both adaptive and maladaptive coping strategies than youth who do not (Trepal et al., 2015). This means that when these youth are under stress, they are likely moving from strategy to strategy in a frantic attempt to de-escalate on their own (Wester et al., 2017). Clearly, students who self-injure may know about healthy coping strategies but have difficulty applying them in the moment. Helping them slow down, be intentional, and stay with one strategy long enough for it to actually begin to work is important. It is for this reason that a mindfulness-based approach may be especially promising for students who self-injure.*

Teaching and Staff In-Service Training

There is a clear need for training of school personnel on students and self-injury. Unfortunately, most school staff have not been trained on the topic, and even among school mental health professionals, three-quarters say they have not received any education or training on NSSI (Kelada et al., 2017).

All school personnel should receive periodic trainings on NSSI, including what it is, how to identify and respond to it, how to help students develop healthy coping strategies, and, most importantly, how to help students access appropriate help. As staff are trained, it is important to help them learn how to take a nonjudgmental stance when engaging with students who self-injure. Although NSSI behavior can be disturbing, it is important to approach the student's behavior calmly and with a caring attitude.

Teachers and other staff who are not trained as mental health professionals are an extremely important link in the chain. Helping these staff members recognize how to encourage and support the student and assist with follow-through to appropriate services within the school is the most important outcome of these types of in-service trainings. Teachers need to know that it is *not their role* to stop NSSI, but rather to help identify and refer students they suspect of engaging in NSSI to the designated school mental health professional (e.g., school counselor, school psychologist, nurse, or administrator). Teachers and other staff who provide these referrals also can provide critical information concerning the student's interactions with peers; clues or warning signs presented in the student's schoolwork, such as artwork or writing; and other behavioral observations.

Just as important as it is to know what to do, it is important to help teachers and others in the school know what *not to do* with a youth exhibiting NSSI behaviors. It is important not to shame or guilt the student or to discuss the student's self-harming behaviors in front of peers, even if the student initiates those conversations in front of others. Further, no matter the circumstances, school staff and teachers should *never* collude with a student regarding NSSI behavior or make deals with a student to get them to stop. These types of negotiations are sometimes tempting, but they are *always* inappropriate. Students may plead with teachers to keep their NSSI behavior secret, but this request *cannot* be fulfilled. Finally, the use of punishment or other negative consequences if the student self-injures is never an appropriate response.

As with all school policies, the time to develop how to handle any potentially harmful situation, including NSSI, is before the situation presents itself. As you read this, stop and think about your own school for a moment. If possible, talk with colleagues and school administrators about the current policies, training, and intervention approaches concerning NSSI in your school. Is there a need to develop some prevention programming and training? Chances are there is work that needs to be done. Most schools have very limited written policies and procedures for working with these students. A proactive approach to developing and disseminating a school-wide policy and procedure for working with these students will benefit everyone at the school.

> *Practical strategy (schools): National studies find that most schools do not have a policy about how to respond to students who engage in NSSI, and most staff are unsure of whether such a policy exists in their school (Kelada et al., 2017). Therefore, an important first step is the development of a school-wide policy and dissemination of that policy to all staff in the school. Topics that should be addressed within that policy include (SIOutReach.org, 2018):*
> * *Describe the warning signs that may signal a student has self-injured.*
> * *Outline how school staff should initially respond when they believe a student has self-injured.*
> * *Clearly define when school staff should report a student they suspect of self-injuring.*
> * *Clearly state to whom school staff should report students who self-injure (or are suspected of self-injuring).*
> * *Describe what feedback (if any) will be provided to the school staff member who initially referred the student.*
> * *List and clearly define the specific roles and tasks of each member of the school staff in the identification, assessment, reporting, and referral process.*
> * *Describe the specific protocols that will be used for the initial and follow-up risk assessments and who is responsible for conducting these.*
> * *Describe whether, when, and how to notify parents/guardians.*
> * *Describe when a student should be referred to outside services.*
> * *Describe when a student should be referred to emergency mental health services.*
> * *Decide a school policy regarding ongoing parent contact.*

- *Detail how to limit contagion among other students. For example, the policy might include clear guidance about how to ask students to cover existing new wounds. This should include balancing a student's desire to conceal or not conceal wounds with the potential that these could create triggering conditions for other students at risk. This plan should also include a discussion for transition to revealing scars when the student expresses a wish to do so, with the recognition that this may signal a positive step in the student's recovery. This must be coupled with both a plan for protecting other vulnerable students and a plan for alerting appropriate school personnel if the student is bullied due to the scars. Regular check-ins must occur.*

Lowering the Risk of Contagion. There is real concern that NSSI can be contagious among groups of students in school, and that risk can be heightened after exposure in the media, over the Internet, or by the self-harming behaviors of a classmate. Anecdotal reports tell us that many children who self-injure first get the idea from a friend or the media. We have seen first-hand how self-injury can sweep through a vulnerable population. One of us worked with high-risk teens in a day treatment facility for survivors of severe trauma. Although there had been a history of self-injury among some of the teens, there was no current NSSI among any members. One day, a young woman came into group with severe cuts on her arm. The next day, another woman had cuts. Within days, every member of the group, including those with no history of NSSI, had lacerations to their hands, arms, legs, and breasts. In spite of the winter weather in the northern climate, members of the group wore tank tops and shorts to group, even though just days earlier they wore sweaters and jeans. Within a week, it had become the norm for members of the group to self-injure and to display their fresh wounds with pride.

Although there is certainly reason for caution, the actual risk of contagion among school-aged children is unclear. It is possible that discussions of self-harm or displays of another student's scars could be triggering for a student who is at risk, and it is for this reason that most schools have policies against open discussions of NSSI and require students with open self-inflicted wounds to cover them.

> *Practical strategy (schools): All of the available research and writing about NSSI tells us that the most important strategy to limit contagion is to stop students from talking about self-injury. In fact, most guidelines simply state, "Do not allow students to share detailed information regarding their self-injury, to share images, or to share stories." If you are like us, you're probably shaking your head right now—maybe even laughing at the naivete of that statement. We know from experience that it's pretty tough—or downright impossible—to stop teenagers from sharing stories or pictures that they want to share. So, what can we do? Well, first and foremost, <u>we can stop sharing</u>. Don't use school-wide assemblies, newsletters, or other media to address an "outbreak" of NSSI. Don't use group counseling or other group interventions to manage self-injury. Groups can lead to one-upmanship and exacerbation. Never discuss a student's self-injury in front of their peers or other school staff, even if they start the conversation in public. Finally, our experience is that if we help students to understand why engaging in conversations about NSSI with their peers is dangerous, many of them will stop—or at least limit their behaviors. Although many seek attention for themselves, we have learned that many do not want this for others. They may be intent on harming themselves, but when they understand how their behaviors might harm others who might be at risk, they often (not always, but often) stop.*

Assessment and Referral

The primary responsibility of the school mental health professional is to assess and appropriately refer a youth who has been identified as engaging in NSSI behavior. A clinical assessment for

NSSI requires advanced training and is not something that is generally done within the school system. In general, these types of assessments include (a) medical history, (b) substance use history, (c) identification of possible comorbid mental health diagnoses, (d) evaluation of risk and preventative factors, and (e) evaluation of family and other social supports (Walsh, 2006). Certainly the medical assessment and evaluation must be completed by an individual who has the appropriate medical credentials, whether this is done by a school nurse or someone in an external medical setting (Stargell et al., 2017). Within schools, the type of risk assessment that is completed by school mental health professionals is generally less clinical and more functional. Unless the student is in obvious emotional distress that requires emergency care or has physical wounds that require attention, an assessment should include both the physical aspects of the self-injury (e.g., "Where on your body do you typically self-injure?"; "Have you ever hurt yourself more seriously than you intended?") as well as the nonphysical (emotional, cognitive, social, environmental) antecedents to the self-harm (e.g., "What were you feeling/thinking before you engaged in the behavior?"; "What happened right before you engaged in the behavior?"). Because of the uncertain link between NSSI and suicide (discussed below), a risk assessment for NSSI should always include a risk assessment for suicide (see Stargell et al., 2017 for a list of specific questions for school counselors to guide assessments).

As school mental health professionals reach out to family members, remember that students who self-injure, *in general*, perceive that they have poorer relationships with their parents and receive higher levels of criticism, less support, greater psychological control, and higher levels of family-based loneliness than students who do not self-injure (Whitlock et al., 2018). Therefore, these initial contacts with parents and guardians can be particularly challenging. Nevertheless, these difficult relationships that often exist between these students and their parents and guardians underscore the importance of the role of the family in helping these students recover.

> *Practical strategy (schools): We know that it can be difficult to reach out to parents when their child is exhibiting self-harming behaviors. Perhaps understandably, parents can have reactions that make a collaborative relationship between the school and the parent challenging. We hear time and again from school counselors or school psychologists that when they try to tell parents that their child is suffering, their words are met with anger, silence, or tears. Nevertheless, it is the role of the school mental health professional to facilitate this collaborative relationship on behalf of the student. We encourage you to consider what it is like to be a parent in this situation. Perhaps you have seen your child's behaviors and haven't known what to do. Now the school is calling, and you feel guilty or ashamed—like your parenting skills (or lack thereof) are being called into question. Perhaps you are worried that the school will "call the authorities"—and you will have to defend yourself to someone else. Maybe you are angry. With yourself? With your child? It's best to take a deep breath and try to use all your skills to align with the parent right from the start. Bubrick et al. (2010) recommend these strategies:*
>
> * *What if the parent feels guilty? A parent who feels guilty may be feeling inadequate. It may be helpful to offer them resources or remind them that they might need counseling for themselves to get through this difficult time.*
> * *What if the parent is dismissive? The role of the school remains the same: to encourage the parent to be responsive to the child's needs.*
> * *What if the parent has an extreme emotional reaction? Again, the role of the school is to encourage the parent to try to understand the child's needs, to recognize that the child is suffering and would benefit from outside counseling, and to remain calm and nonjudgmental.*

A Note About Therapeutic Interventions With Students Who Self-Harm. Although this chapter is not designed to teach school mental health professionals how to do therapeutic interventions with students who engage in self-injury, we believe that having a basic understanding of the clinical therapeutic process can help school professionals be allies in a student's clinical care. For that reason, we will provide a *very brief* overview of the current state of clinical practice, with the understanding that research in this area moves quickly. In addition, each student's clinical needs differ. Therefore, to be true allies in a student's mental health care, it is essential that school mental health professionals have appropriate releases signed with a student's off-site providers so that everyone can work together in the best interest of the student.

Most clinical interventions are effective but produce small reductions in self-harm that are, in general, maintained over time. To date, no interventions have been found to be consistently better than others (Fox et al., 2020), and in most cases, treatment for NSSI is provided in outpatient settings, as long as the student can be safe. Standard practice is often Dialectical Behavior Therapy (DBT), which is considered a well-established treatment for NSSI. Some clinicians also use Cognitive Behavioral Therapy (CBT; either individually or individual plus family). Finally, mentalization-based therapy, which encourages clients to think more intentionally about their own and others' mental states and awareness of the self, can be an adjunctive treatment (Elmaghraby et al., 2019). The point is, school mental health professionals who wish to be supportive of students who are receiving off-campus mental health care can best achieve this by working with the students' mental health providers and supporting the treatment goals when students are in the school building.

Practical strategy (schools): Safety plans can help students who self-injure develop positive strategies to help them when they have the urge to self-harm. These plans <u>should only be developed with</u>

the assistance of mental health professionals. They are intended to offer short- and medium-term options to help get students through these difficult moments. They should be short (no longer than a page) and include (a) reasons the student has developed for wanting to be healthy/safe; (b) strategies for making the environment safe; (c) warning signs that the student is escalating/triggers; (d) "on my own" coping or strategies for distraction; (e) "with someone" coping strategies, including family and friends; (f) how to tell someone else; (g) names and contact information of the people they will tell; and (h) crisis information. Students should have this information with them at all times. We recommend that they take a picture of the safety plan so they always have it accessible in their phones.

The Uncertain Link Between NSSI and Suicide

No one is absolutely certain about the link between NSSI and suicide. Some believe that because the motivations behind NSSI appear to be different than the motivations behind suicide, they are unrelated. Others say that NSSI helps create a release valve for extreme negative emotions, which can actually lower suicide risk. Still others argue that once the biological imperative not to harm oneself is breached, it becomes easier and easier to engage in those behaviors in the future. From that perspective, NSSI becomes a "gateway drug" to more extreme methods of self-harm, including suicide attempts. We think the reason there is no clear consensus is because there are many different reasons that young people engage in self-injury as well as many different pathways to suicide. For this reason, we are skeptical of any blanket statements about the link between NSSI and suicide. We advise you to take care as you read the following pages. Remember that *any individual student can follow a unique pathway.*

In general, about a third of young people who engage in NSSI report at least some level of current or past suicidality, although it is difficult to fully understand exactly what they mean when they respond "yes" to survey questions about suicidal thoughts or behaviors and how these are connected to their current self-harm. Part of the challenge, of course, is that many of the risk factors for both NSSI and suicide are the same (e.g., history of trauma, limited coping skills, high levels of depression and/or anxiety, isolation or withdrawal, substance use, feelings of worthlessness). Nevertheless, there are some factors that appear to put young people who engage in NSSI at higher risk for also having suicidal thoughts or behaviors. These are high levels of impulsivity, chronic engagement in rNSSI (over 20 lifetime incidents of significant events), high psychological distress during the last month, history of trauma, hopelessness, family conflict and dysfunction, substance use, and a diagnosis of either depression or posttraumatic stress disorder (Whitlock et al., 2015).

Both Suicide and NSSI Are About Psychological Pain. Students Just See Different Outcomes . Students who are suicidal and students who engage in NSSI, in general, both are in tremendous psychological pain. Students who engage in suicidal behaviors (thoughts, planning, attempts) are looking for a way to *end the intense pain,* and they believe that the way to do that is through death, or planning for death. Students who engage in NSSI are seeking a strategy to *cope with the intense* psychological pain, and they believe that self-harm will help relieve the pain. It may seem like semantics, but it is an important distinction. Students who are suicidal get to a point when they engage in a very specific, usually infrequent attempt with high lethality. They want to end pain. Students who engage in NSSI often have ongoing self-harm, with low lethality, as a way to manage and cope with their pain on an ongoing basis. They do not believe that the result of their self-injury will be death or the end of the emotional pain. Their self-injury will be just one more moment in their ongoing journey. They believe that their self-injury will generate positive emotions and make them feel better. Consider the contrast. It is not a perceived endpoint, like it is for students who are preparing for a suicide attempt. As a result, these students often differ in their cognitive states. Students who are suicidal often appear more hopeless and helpless with less of a vision of the future than students who engage in NSSI.

Practical strategy (parents): When parents learn their child is engaging in self-harm, finding appropriate mental health care is critical. Parents who are educated about self-harm in general (e.g., understanding underlying triggers, including the role of negative emotions), as well as their child's own history with self-harm and suicidal thoughts and behaviors (if any), will have a greater likelihood of finding an appropriate therapeutic placement for their child (Fox et al., 2020). We tell parents that it may take meeting with several different therapists or going to several different agencies or treatment centers to find the right "fit" for your child. This is important because a strong therapeutic alliance is one of the best predictors of success for mental health outcomes.

Conclusion

In any school building, there are significant numbers of students who engage in NSSI. Identifying these students, contacting parents, and getting the students to appropriate care—all without encouraging contagion—is the appropriate role of the school mental health professionals. The motivations for self-injury differ by student, and the link between self-injury and suicide is unclear (and also differs by student). Nevertheless, the risk that these behaviors can escalate (even unintentionally) to serious injury as well as the clear evidence that these students are suffering from underlying psychological distress means that these behaviors must be taken seriously and the students must receive appropriate mental health care.

References

Bubrick, K., Goodman, J., & Whitlock, J. (2010). *Non-suicidal self-injury in schools: Developing & implementing school protocol.* The Information Brief Series, Cornell Research Program on Self-Injury and Recovery. Cornell University.

Centers for Disease Control and Prevention (CDC). (2019). *Youth Risk Behavior Surveillance System (YRBSS) 2019.* https://www.cdc.gov/healthyyo uth/data/yrbs/index.htm

Cerutti, R., Calabrese, M., & Valastro, C. (2014). Alexithymia and personality disorders in the adolescent non-suicidal self-injury: Preliminary results. *Procedía—Social and Behavioral Sciences, 114,* 372–376. https://doi.org/10.1016/j.sbspro.2013.12.714

DeCamp, W., & Bakken, N. W. (2016). Self-injury, suicide ideation, and sexual orientation: Differences in causes and correlates among high school students. *Journal of Injury and Violence Research, 8*(1), 15–24.

Elmaghraby, R., Nobari, O., & Cullen, K. R. (2019). Treatment of Non-Suicidal Self-Injurious behavior in adolescents. *Psychiatric Times, 36*(11), 39–42.

Fox, K. R., Huang, X., Guzmán, E. M., Funsch, K. M., Cha, C. B., Ribeiro, J. D., & Franklin, J. C. (2020). Interventions for suicide and self-injury: A meta-analysis of randomized controlled trials across nearly 50 years of research. *Psychological Bulletin, 146*(12), 1117–1145. DOI:10.1037/bul0000305

Gratz, K. L., & Romer, L. (2004). Multidimensional assessment of emotion regulation and dysregulation: Development, factor structure and initial validation of the difficulties in emotion regulation scale. *Journal of Psychopathology & Behavioral Assessment, 26*(4), 41–54.

Green, J. D., & Jakupak, M. (2016). Masculinity and men's self harm behaviors: Implications for non-suicidal self-injury disorder. *Psychology of Men & Masculinity, 17,* 147–155.

Kelada, L., Hasking, P., & Melvin, G. A. (2017). School response to self-injury: Concerns of mental health staff and parents. *School Psychology Quarterly, 32*(2), 173–187.

Meerwijk, E. L., Ford, J. M., & Weiss, S. J. (2013). Brain regions associated with psychological pain: Implications for a neural network and its relationship to physical pain. *Brain Imaging and Behavior, 7*(1), 1–14. doi:10.1007/s11682-012-9179-y

Muehlenkamp, J. J., Walsh, B. W., & McDade, M. (2010). Preventing non-suicidal self-injury in adolescents: The Signs of Self Injury program. *Journal of Youth & Adolescence, 39,* 306–314.

Muehlenkamp, J. J., Xhunga, N., & Brausch, A. M. (2018). Self-injury age of onset: A risk factor for NSSI severity and suicidal behavior. *Archives of Suicide Research, 23*(4), 551–563. doi:10.1080/13811118.2018.1486252

NYC Health. (2017). Stressors, mental health, and sources of support among LGBTQ public high school students in New York City. *Epi Data Brief, 93.* https://www1.nyc.gov/assets/doh/downloads/pdf/epi/databrief93.pdf

SIOutReach.org. (2018). *Self-injury: A guide for school professionals.* University of Guelph & McGill University. http://sioutreach.org/learn-self-injury/school-professionals/

Sornberger, M., Heath, N., Toste, N., & McLouth, R. (2012). Nonsuicidal self-injury and gender: Patterns of prevalence, methods, and locations among adolescents. *Suicide & Life-Threatening Behavior, 42,* 266–278. doi:10.1111/j.1943-278X.2012.0088.x

Stargell, N. A., Zoldan, C. A., Kress, V. E., Walker-Andrews, L. M., & Whisenhunt, J. L. (2017). Student non-suicidal self-injury: A protocol for school counselors. *Professional School Counseling, 21*(1), 37–46.

Störkel, L. M., Karabatsiakis, A., Hepp, J., Kolassa, I-T., Schmahl, C., & Niedtfeld, I. (2021). Salivary beta-endorphin in nonsuicidal self-injury: An ambulatory assessment study. *Neuropsychopharmacology, 46*(7), 1357–1363. doi:10.1038/s41386-020-00914-2

Trepal, H. C., Wester, K. L., & Merchant, E. (2015). A cross sectional matched sample study of non-suicidal self-injury among young adults: Support for interpersonal and intrapersonal factors, with implications for coping strategies. *Child and Adolescent Psychiatry and Mental Health, 9,* 36. https://doi.org/10.1186/s13034-015-0070-7

Walsh, B. W. (2006). *Treating self-injury: A practical guide.* Guilford.

Wester, K. L., Morris, C. W., & Williams, B. (2017). NSSI in the schools: A tiered prevention approach for reducing social contagion. *Professional School Counseling, 21,* 142–151.

Westers, N. J., Lewis, S. P., Whitlock, J., Schatten, H. T., Ammerman, B., Andover, M. S., & Lloyd-Richardson, E. E. (2021). Media guidelines for the responsible reporting and depicting of non-suicidal self-injury. *The British Journal of Psychiatry, 219*(2), 1–4. doi:10.1192/bjp.2020.191

Whitlock, J. (2018). *Understanding adolescent self-injury* [Lecture PowerPoint]. http://www.selfinjury.bctr.cornell.edu/

Whitlock, J., Baetens, I., Lloyd-Richardson, E., Hasking, P., Hamza, C., Lewis, S., Franz, P., & Robinson, K. (2018). Helping schools support caregivers of youth who self-injure: Considerations and recommendations. *School Psychology International, 39*(3), 312–328. doi:10.1177/0143034318771415

Whitlock, J., Minton, R., Babington, P., & Ernhout, C. (2015). *The relationship between non-suicidal self-injury and suicide.* The Information Brief Series, Cornell Research Program on Self-Injury and Recovery. Cornell University.

You, J., Ren, Y., Zhang, X., Wu, Z., Xu, S., & Lin, M-P. (2018). Emotional dysregulation and nonsuicidal self-injury: A meta-analytic review. *Neuropsychiatry, 8*(2), 733–748.

6

Building the Foundation of a School-Based Suicide Prevention Program

The nation's schools play an essential role in youth suicide prevention. Clearly, school-based suicide prevention programming has the potential to save the lives of students who may be at risk. In addition, this type of programming can instill the values of mental health help seeking and the prosocial behaviors of how to reach out to others in distress in all young people that can last a lifetime. School-based suicide prevention programs help keep students safe by teaching everyone in the building how to identify risk factors and warning signs as well as how to intervene with at-risk youth. In addition, these programs provide access to information and resources that are responsive to students' personal and social-emotional needs.

At school, students can learn about the role of stigma in mental health, healthy help-seeking behaviors, how to intervene if they believe a friend may be at risk for suicide, how to access care for themselves, and how to develop protective skills that can help minimize their own risk. Students who may be at risk benefit when many people at the school they see and interact with on a daily basis (teachers, counselors, nurses, coaches, staff, and classmates) all have a basic understanding about suicide risk and are confident, competent, and willing to intervene. When suicide prevention programming is part of a larger effort to promote student mental health, the results can be dramatic (e.g., Katz et al., 2013). Unfortunately, without suicide prevention programming and education, schools can become places where students keep secrets, teachers are

Suicide and Self-Injury in Schools. Darcy Haag Granello, Paul F. Granello, Gerald A. Juhnke,
Oxford University Press. © Oxford University Press 2023. DOI: 10.1093/oso/9780190059842.003.0006

uncertain about what to say or do if they see problem behaviors in their students, and common myths and misunderstandings about suicide become the norm.

In spite of recent attention to the problem of child and adolescent suicide, many schools are reluctant to engage in comprehensive suicide prevention programming. At least in part, this reluctance is based on some common myths that often exist within school systems.

- MYTH: Suicide prevention has no place in schools.
  - FACT: Our nation's schools, in partnership with communities and families, are the obvious places to identify suicidal youth and to provide information to all children and their families. School personnel are a key population to receive knowledge and training in suicide prevention, as outlined in the 2012 National Strategy for Suicide Prevention (U.S. Department of Health & Human Services, 2012). Other national organizations, such as the American Foundation for Suicide Prevention (AFSP) and the Jed Foundation, also specifically feature the importance of training school personnel in suicide prevention. Although there are many reasons schools are identified as the primary place for youth suicide prevention, the primary reasons include the following:
    - Maintaining a safe school environment is part of a school's overall mission.
    - In schools, students spend time with their peers, meaning that problems they may have with interpersonal functioning may be more evident than at home or in the community.
    - Because of the amount of time students spend in schools, students who are struggling with suicidal behaviors are likely to exhibit these behaviors during school hours.

- In schools, students have access to many different individuals, meaning that there is a higher likelihood that trained individuals will recognize that there are problems and intervene.
- If students feel connected to their schools or to people in their schools (e.g., they believe that teachers, staff, or other students care about them), they may be more likely to reach out for assistance or even less likely to engage in suicidal behaviors.
- Schools are appropriate places to serve the holistic health and wellness needs of children. A whole-child approach to education recognizes that a student's physical and emotional health is integral to educational outcomes.
- The needs of all students are best managed through a co-ordinated approach, such as one in a school-based suicide prevention program.

- MYTH: My professional association does not think I should get involved in school-based suicide prevention.
  - FACT: The professional associations of the school-based mental health and administrative professions have taken a strong stand to promote the role of its members as advocates for student mental health and suicide prevention. Each of these professions has endorsed strong policy statements *while simultaneously reminding its members* of the importance of training and professional ethics around this important topic. In other words, members of these professions are reminded that they have an important role to play, within the boundaries and scope of their professional training and ethics. You can check out the position of your professional association here.
    - School counselors
      - The American School Counselor Association (ASCA) has endorsed a *Model School District Policy on Suicide*

Prevention that includes information about the appropriate role of the school counselor as a leader in this effort. It is available on their website (http://www.scho olcounselor.org).

- School psychologists
  - The National Association of School Psychologists (NASP) has endorsed a *Model School District Policy on Suicide Prevention* that includes information about the appropriate role of the school psychologist as a leader in this effort. It is available on their website (http://www.nasp.org).
- School nurses
  - The National Association of School Nurses (NASN) has a position statement on the *Behavioral Health and Wellness of Students*, which recognizes the importance of school nurses as essential to suicide prevention, because they are often the first to recognize and address the behavioral health concerns of students (https:// www.nasn.org).
- School social workers
  - The School Social Worker Association of America (SSWAA) states that their unique mission is to provide the link between the school and the community, with specific attention given to students in mental health crisis (http://www.sswaa.org).
- School principals
  - The National Association of Secondary School Principals (NASSP) has a position statement on the *Mental Health of Middle and High School Students,* including the importance of suicide prevention, with a clear role articulated for school principals and other administrative leaders (http://www.nassp.org).
- MYTH: Talking about suicide in schools will put the idea in students' heads.

- FACT: This is a particularly dangerous myth. Spreading this myth is not only irresponsible but also actually harmful to students and to school-wide suicide prevention efforts.
  - The reality is that talking about suicide and suicidal thoughts and feelings can greatly reduce the distress that suicidal people feel. Talking to people about suicide helps them understand that we care—that they are not alone.
  - We understand that school administrators are often worried that somehow if they allow suicide prevention programs in their schools, they will inadvertently unleash a spate of suicidal behavior. However, research *consistently* finds that when suicide is discussed appropriately in school-based suicide prevention programming, increases in suicidal behavior *do not occur*. In fact, school-based suicide prevention programming lowers suicide risk for students. A large-scale national study comparing schools that had suicide prevention programs to those that did not found that *overall*, there were fewer student deaths in schools with suicide prevention programs (Walrath et el., 2015).
  - Another study of more than 2,000 adolescents found depressed teenagers were *not more likely* to consider suicide after it was brought up in a class. In fact, depressed teenagers who had attempted suicide in the past reported that they were *less likely* to be suicidal or upset after the discussion (Gould et al., 2005).
  - Additionally, there are more than 30 years of crisis hotline experience and more than 25 years of school-based suicide prevention programming with *not one single documented case of stimulating suicidal behavior through discussion of the topic.*
  - The fact is, we don't give people the idea of suicide simply by bringing up the topic. Rather, we give people permission to talk about their suicidal thoughts and feelings in

appropriate ways, to learn how to seek help, and to find ways other than suicide to manage their unbearable pain.

- MYTH: Schools can be sued if they have a suicide prevention program.
  - FACT: Actually, the opposite is true. Schools can be successfully sued if they ignore this important component of student life. In fact, two important court cases set legal precedent for the role of schools in suicide prevention. In *Kelson v. the City of Springfield, Oregon* (1985), a judge ruled that an inadequate response of the school staff resulted in the death of a 14-year-old student. This case established the precedent that parents of a student who completes suicide can *sue the school* if the death allegedly resulted from inadequate school-based prevention. Further, the findings in this case demanded that *all school staff* (e.g., janitors, lunchroom personnel, secretaries), not just teachers and administrators, are responsible for protection of the student.
  - In the second case, *Wyke v. Polk County School Board* (1997), the court found that a school that did not have a fully developed suicide prevention policy in place was negligent when it failed to notify parents of suicide attempts of a 13-year-old student. The judgment in this case is significant because it indicates that school administrators and teachers can be held liable for not recognizing and reporting a student who is at risk for suicide, which has clear implications for staff training in suicide risk.
  - Currently, there are no federal laws that require schools to provide suicide prevention programming for their students, faculty, and staff. However, a model state law, called the Jason Flatt Act, requires all K–12 educators to receive 2 hours of in-service awareness and prevention training *each year* to remain licensed. In 2009, Tennessee was the first state to pass the Jason Flatt Act. As of 2022, 21 states have signed this Act into law. You can check here to see if your

state has signed this Act into law and to learn how to advocate for this legislation if it has not: https://jasonfoundation.
com/about-us/jason-flatt-act/.

- In addition, although not all states have laws that require
  the level of training required by the Jason Flatt Act, 46 states
  have laws that address either student or staff education on
  suicide (Smith-Millman & Flaspohler, 2019).
- MYTH: Suicide programs lead to contagion and "copycat"
  suicides.
  - FACT: Copycat suicides do exist, and if someone is al-
    ready vulnerable (e.g., depressed, showing warning signs,
    has made a previous attempt), then one suicide in a school
    system can trigger another. However, it is not the school-
    based suicide prevention programming that leads to cop-
    ycat suicides—it is the existence of other completed suicides
    in a young person's life (either in the school system, in the
    media, or elsewhere in the community). Thus, primary pre-
    vention programming is intended to mitigate the *already
    existing danger* of copycat suicides in the schools.

These myths (and others) can have serious negative consequences
for the school climate. In our work with schools, we often find that
there are local myths or rumors that have developed over time
(often loosely based in a story or gossip). We have found that it is
important to understand these local stories because they are often
extremely powerful and have great potential to do damage. All of
these myths underscore the importance of a fact-based school-
based suicide prevention program to help promote a healthier
environment.

*Practical strategy (schools): Whenever possible, we encourage
the people who are engaging in the initial planning to do a little
investigating. What are the local stories? What are the specific
myths? The "urban legends"? Of course, they may not be true—or*

they may be loosely true or based in old stories. Nevertheless, these rumors and stories often hold power. Knowing any local myths or rumors that will need to be "undone" through the school-based program (keeping in mind that many of the stories cannot be addressed directly, due to Family Educational Rights and Privacy Act (FERPA) and Health Insurance Portability and Accountability Act (HIPAA) concerns) can be helpful.

Levels of School-Based Prevention

Anyone who works in a school is probably at least somewhat familiar with the three tiers of prevention programming (Gordon, 1987), and suicide prevention follows this general approach. Each tier addresses a different population and has a different purpose (Figure 6.1).

Typically, Comprehensive School-Based Suicide Prevention Programming in schools starts with an approach that is directed at the entire population in the school. This tier one approach is called **universal prevention**. The goal of universal prevention is to make sure everyone within the system (students, staff, teachers,

The Three Tiers of Prevention Programming

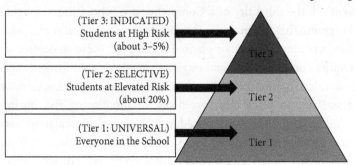

Figure 6.1 The Three Tiers of Prevention Programming

and parents) has some basic understanding and awareness regarding suicide risk, including warning signs, risk factors, how to ask for help, and how to respond to a potentially suicidal student or peer. Universal prevention also typically includes efforts to reduce stigma for mental health help seeking, generic coping skills, and other protective factors, such as strategies to build a sense of connection and community within the school.

When prevention strategies are focused on segments of the population that are characterized by certain risk factors, this tier two approach is called **selective prevention/intervention**. This is done with students who are already identified as potentially at risk for suicide because they have poor coping skills, for example, or because they have experienced a loss by suicide or have some other characteristic or experience that places them at risk. Students in this category will undoubtedly need more assistance than the education provided through the universal intervention program. These students might need individual or group counseling to help them improve their coping skills or resilience, assistance with accessing community resources, or more specific screening or assessment. These types of intervention strategies will be discussed in Chapters 8 and 9.

Finally, there are students who require specific individual assistance because they have been specifically identified as at risk for suicide. These students require **indicated prevention/intervention**, the third tier of a Comprehensive School-Based Suicide Program. This tier provides individual assistance to students who have suicidal thoughts or plans. For example, these students may require comprehensive and ongoing suicide risk assessments and referrals to community resources. To assist these students, schools must have in place clear protocols for monitoring risk during school hours, established procedures for managing escalation, and strategies for open and ongoing communication between school personnel, parents, and mental health providers. Indicated intervention strategies will be discussed in Chapters 8 and 9.

The Overall School-Based Suicide Prevention and Intervention Plan

We believe it is important for everyone involved in suicide prevention programming to understand the big picture for suicide prevention, intervention, and postvention, even though tier 2 and 3 intervention and postvention are not typically strategies that will be discussed and developed by the Core Team as they create a suicide prevention plan for the school. Nevertheless, we find it is helpful to have a conceptual model to help everyone involved understand the big picture and how their role fits into that approach. Toward that end, we typically offer this model to aid in that understanding.

The Comprehensive School-Based Suicide Prevention Model

There are 10 major components to a comprehensive school-based approach to working with suicidal students (Figure 6.2). The first

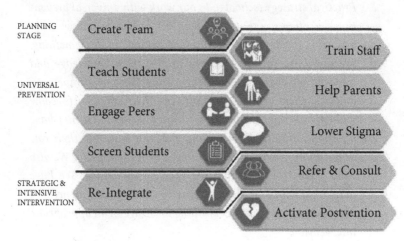

Figure 6.2 A Comprehensive Model for School-Based Suicide Prevention

(planning stage) and the six listed next to "universal prevention" in Figure 6.2 are in the realm of prevention. They are the focus of this chapter and the next.

Three elements of the model—listed next to "selective & indicated intervention in Figure 6.2—and under the last line of the model—are approaches that are primarily appropriate for students who are already identified as suicidal or are part of the crisis response plan for the school after a suicide has occurred. These three components are NOT considered part of prevention planning and will be discussed in subsequent chapters.

In this chapter, we turn our attention to the first tier of a comprehensive approach: universal intervention. The goal is to promote a climate where all students, staff, teachers, and parents have information about suicide, understand their role in helping to prevent suicide, and believe that they can do something to help. This is how we help change the culture in a school. This is how we lower the stigma of help seeking. It all starts here.

> *Practical strategy (schools): In our work with universal prevention, we often say that it is about helping the people we train become "confident, competent, and willing" to do something. We use universal interventions to give them knowledge and information (become confident), skills (become competent), and help them change—or reinforce—their attitudes (become willing). We want the people we train to believe that they have a responsibility to do something, that this is part of their role as a staff or faculty member (or even as student peers. We also want them to believe that they can do something. We have found that with proper education and training (confidence and competence), they are more willing to engage in an appropriate intervention.*

A Broad-Based Approach to School-Based Suicide Prevention: A Step-by-Step Guide to the Process

In general, a Comprehensive School-Based Suicide Prevention Program relies on a broad-based approach to meet the needs of the students. There is no universally agreed-upon program for schools to implement, nor is there an evidence-based best practice model that is currently available. There is, however, general agreement that a school-wide approach that involves a collaborative team effort works best.

In this section of the chapter, we will focus on laying the foundation for a school-based prevention program. This type of programming doesn't just happen, and it certainly isn't something that one individual in the building should implement without support and buy-in from the school administrators, staff, teachers, and, when possible, parents and the larger community. It may be frustrating to take time to be thoughtful, careful, and planful about each step of the planning process, especially when it can feel like there is pressure to do something *now* because students are hurting *now*. However, we have found that when it comes to suicide prevention programming, acting quickly is simply not a good idea. We have seen well-intentioned suicide prevention programs fail when others in the school building weren't consulted. We have seen those who felt excluded sabotage the work, believing that their ideas and strategies were better and should have been implemented instead. We have seen people with great intentions speak to students about suicide in ways that, at best, probably did very little to help and, at worst, may have escalated suicidal behaviors in some of the students. Finally, we have seen large and time-consuming suicide prevention programs land at the feet of a single staff person who became quickly overwhelmed and exhausted, with the result that you might expect: a great program that no longer exists.

However, we have also seen comprehensive school-based programs that are successful, long-lasting, and effective. The common feature of all of the successful programs is a thoughtful foundation with a strategic plan that involves a team of leaders who share a common vision. In the next pages, we will help you create that foundation in your school building. We have trained many schools and districts in this model, and a consistent piece of feedback from the teams we train is summed up in the words of one participant: "This brings to light that we have to have a more concrete plan. We know this is important, but we somehow haven't gotten around to it. I guess we didn't know where to start. This model finally gave us the tools." We hope that the model will give you these tools to begin your comprehensive plan too.

Step 1: Create a Core Team

In any school building, there will be a core group of staff and administrators who shepherd the suicide prevention program from initial development through implementation. Typically, these are the staff who would normally be involved in the care of at-risk students. If you are reading this book, chances are *you are one of those people*. The Core Team is typically interdisciplinary. It often consists of school mental health professionals, such as school counselors, school psychologists, school social workers, nurses, and school resource officers. The team also might include administrators, such as principals or others in the building who are self-identified advocates who have expressed a specific interest in suicide prevention. Core Teams might include coaches, educators from major academic areas, or other specific individuals who are appropriate for an individual school. The Core Team should be small enough to be flexible for planning purposes (perhaps five to eight key individuals), with the recognition that there will be room for a larger planning group in the next stage.

In some school districts, suicide prevention is not done at the individual school level, but there is a more coordinated district-wide effort. The AFSP *Model School District Policy on Suicide Prevention* (2019) recommends that each school district have a Suicide Prevention Coordinator who helps oversee the suicide prevention work done in the individual school buildings within the district. Ideally, this district coordinator would interact with the school's Core Team to ensure a consistent, district-wide effort. We recognize that this may or may not be the case in your school. You may have a district-wide Suicide Prevention Coordinator who is overseeing the work in the schools. (*You may even be this person. Congratulations. You are __way__ ahead of most school districts if you are!*) If not, and if you don't have a coordinated district policy, the school-based Core Team can still move forward—and perhaps agree to reach out to other schools within your district to work together, as appropriate.

In each school, the Core Team typically has one person who coordinates the effort and becomes that building's Suicide Prevention Coordinator. This is typically an existing staff person, who is often a mental health professional. The Core Team meets initially for members to express interest and develop a preliminary strategy.

Practical strategy (schools): Create a new team. Although there is clearly overlap between this team and a multitude of other teams that already exist in the school (e.g., teams on violence prevention, mental health, Positive Behavioral Interventions and Supports (PBIS), and a multitude of other initiatives), we caution you not to use an existing team and simply "tack on" suicide prevention as another project. We have seen this before, and what we have seen is that suicide prevention simply gets lost among the multitude of other responsibilities and priorities. Unless there is a team specifically devoted to suicide prevention, with timelines, goals, and priorities, it is too easy to have this work drop to the bottom of already crowded agendas.

Ultimately, as the Core Team moves forward, they will be the ones who build, oversee, and champion the plan (Jed Foundation, 2021). However, we always caution this team not to make too many plans or move too far into all of the details of the process before they move to step 2, administrative buy-in. Nevertheless, the Core Team will need to have some initial planning meetings and develop an overall vision of what they want to accomplish and what they see as the ultimate goal of their school's prevention program. We have found that a primary outcome of the initial meetings is to generate a commitment for an overall shared vision.

> *Practical strategy (schools): What is the shared vision of the Core Team? We are often surprised when we meet with a team that wants to develop a school-based suicide prevention program for the first time. When we do, it can sometimes become apparent that they <u>think</u> they have a shared vision, but they do not. Some of the team might believe they are working toward a "zero suicide" approach, while others do not believe such a goal is possible. Some might think the goal is to remove students who are suicidal from the school, only allowing them to return when their risk is low, while others think that this messaging prevents students from reaching out. The point is, we often find that people on the team assume that they share the same vision. Taking a few minutes to discuss in some detail what the overarching goal of the program will be is typically well worth the time, builds a unified strategy from the start, and prevents members of the team from sharing contradictory messaging.*

Collect and Use Data to Support the Plan . The Core Team can use existing data to understand the baseline mental health and suicide needs of the students. Existing data might exist, for example, that informs the team about how many students were referred to outside assistance because they were suicidal, how many times parents had been called because of suicidal students, how many students had expressed concerns about their peers, or how often teachers had requested assistance because they were worried that a student might be suicidal. Any school-based data that helps the Core Team as they prepare their overall vision for a school-based prevention program is useful. *However, this type of data is ultimately not what will be used to measure the success of any suicide prevention program. This is the type of data that will be used to help engage the members of the school in this important work.*

If the school does not have existing data, then the national data found in this book can be useful too. After all, there is no particular reason to believe that any individual school's statistics are far removed from the national statistics when it comes to suicide. Extrapolating the national numbers to the local level is a useful way to get a general baseline, with the recognition that each individual school building is unique.

> *Practical strategy (schools): Existing data can be a powerful mechanism to help a Core Team get buy-in from administrators, school boards, and other key players. Data from the school building can also help teachers and staff recognize the magnitude of the problem and the importance of suicide prevention programming. We encourage you to use what you have, even if it is not "scientifically rigorous." In other words, we have found that tick marks in a counselor's daily log that reflect the number of times in a month that a specific counselor consults with teachers about students who might be at risk for suicide are often more compelling than national statistics. Your own students are the reason that others in your building will want to be involved. Tell their story (masked identities, please!)—and then help others understand how a Comprehensive School-Based Suicide Prevention Program can help.*

This is also an opportunity for the Core Team to collect and compile information about what is already in place. In most schools, there are some (often disconnected) efforts around suicide prevention and mental health. It is likely that there are already some aspects of suicide prevention programming (education, advocacy, outreach) going on in your school. Certainly, there is work that is happening with students in crisis (recognizing students in crisis, referral, reintegration after a hospitalization, and postvention).

It's time to take stock of what you have and gather any existing data and information. Here are some questions to get you started:

- What is in place?
- When was the last time education or programming was done? Who did it?
- Who coordinates the suicide prevention efforts?
- Who coordinates the intervention/assessment efforts?
- What policies are in place for postvention?
- Who knows this information?
- What data is available?
- Who has the data?
- Who is able to collect the data on the programming or outreach?
- How will the Core Team collect and use the data?

Step 2: Engage Administrators, School Boards, and Other Key Players

Before any real suicide prevention programming can begin, it is important to gain administrative and stakeholder support (Granello & Zyromski, 2019). It may be necessary and important to include the school superintendent in these discussions, as well as the principal and other school leaders. If there are school advisory boards for student mental health, they also should be included in this step. The point here is to bring together all of the key players to have buy-in and high-level administrative support.

The Core Team should not assume that all of these key players completely understand the magnitude of the problem or the benefits of a Comprehensive School-Based Suicide Prevention Program. Therefore, be prepared to offer a presentation to the key players that highlights the importance of addressing suicide risk among students, the school and national data, and the overall components of a school-based plan that can be used to address the problem. The presentation should also emphasize the groundwork that the Core Team has done, their selection of suicide prevention programs and how these programs are grounded in research and evidence, and how these programs might be generally integrated into the school. We have found that when discussing suicide prevention with key personnel, Core Team members often encounter administrators or board members who have fixed ideas about what types of suicide prevention programming should be offered. Core Team members who are prepared find themselves in a better position to fend off "pet programs or speakers" and to instead base their school's programs in the latest research and evidence.

Practical strategy (schools): Grounding the presentation to key stakeholders in data and evidence while still sharing your passion for helping students is essential. We have found that a few compelling stories (properly masked) that explain why teachers need to recognize warning signs or why students need to know how to ask for help can set an important tone. Then, the national and school-based data help explain the larger picture. When it comes to selecting the types of school-based programs that you might use, we strongly encourage you *to emphasize that although there is no one evidence-based model, everything you do will be grounded in available research and data, and to remind stakeholders that this is essential because of the seriousness of the topic and the danger of contagion if this is handled poorly. We have seen far too many school-based prevention programs highjacked by well-meaning and influential stakeholders who bring in speakers who escalate risk in kids or share outdated material. Having a clear plan when you enter the presentation limits the possibility of this occurring. Then, if a stakeholder suggests "a great speaker that I heard at my church," you have already laid out an evidence-based model that you are following, and that "great speaker who shares their own story" doesn't fit the model. Then, it's up to you to engage the stakeholder who offered the idea in a way that helps them feel important and involved.*

Step 3: Start the Planning Process

Once there is buy-in from the right people, the next step will be gathering data to help fully understand the state of your school. Pre-existing data is helpful, but now is the time for a broader needs assessment. It may be that the Core Team engages in this step *before* they meet with the stakeholders, so that they have more data to share during these important meetings. It may also be that the Core Team holds off on a larger needs assessment about mental health and suicide until after the stakeholders are on board. Regardless of *when* this step is conducted, it is important to get a good understanding of the school's baseline level of functioning.

Make Sure Appropriate Protocols Are in Place. Before any training or education moves out into the larger school community, the Core Team must ensure that there are proper policies, procedures, and protocols in place. This means that there should be procedures and protocols in place for (a) referrals of potentially suicidal students from staff or other students, (b) keeping potentially suicidal students safe during a suicide crisis, (c) interacting with parents (including when there is abuse or neglect at home) and emergency and mental health personnel, (d) reintegration of students after a suicide crisis, and (e) safety planning for suicidal students. (For more information about the types of protocols that should be in place *before* universal education can begin, see Substance Abuse and Mental Health Services Administration [SAMHSA], 2012.)

Collect and Use More Comprehensive Data to Create a Detailed Plan. In step 1, we discussed the use of existing data as an important way to communicate your message to key stakeholders. At this stage, it is probable that the Core Team will want to have more comprehensive data as they develop the details of the comprehensive program. For example, the Core Team may wish to develop and distribute simple questionnaires to teachers about the perceived mental health needs of their students. They might also give students or parents some simple questionnaires about what they think students should learn or know or what they want the school to offer. For example, we are fascinated by the results of a large-scale study, somewhat out of date now, that asked teenagers what they would like to see in school-based suicide prevention programming (Washington County Department of Public Health & Environment, 2001). The results are interesting for several reasons. First, we think that even though the study is rather old, these are still important skills for teens to learn. Second, the scarcity of this type of research reminds us of how seldom we actually ask the students in schools what they need to hear. The teens in this study said they wanted suicide education programming that would:

Teach teens that depression is a form of illness that can be treated	65%
Inform teens how common depression is	56%
Teach teens how to tell if someone is really depressed or just in a mood	68%
Teach teens how to recognize depression in oneself or others	74%
Teach teens where to go for help if they or a friend is depressed or suicidal	73%
Teach teens how to talk to a friend who is depressed or considering suicide	81%

Of course, some schools may wish to engage in a more comprehensive needs assessment. Because the evaluation of a suicide prevention program *should never use suicide as the measure of program success*, now is the time to consider what the Core Team would like to see as a result of the implementation of the suicide prevention program. Perhaps if the model were implemented, students would feel more connected to the school? Maybe they would know how to get help for themselves or their friends? Perhaps the outcome measure would be that they would believe they have learned some important skills in emotional regulation? Whatever it is that the Core Team believes they will accomplish through the program, the needs assessment is a time to gather baseline data. Ideally, the needs assessment should be distributed to all educational stakeholders, including students, staff, teachers, administrators, and parents. The more comprehensive the questionnaires, the clearer the baseline data will be, and the clearer the link between the content offered in the training(s) and the specific needs of the students, staff, and teachers in the school. In addition, clear baseline data can be particularly helpful in determining the effectiveness of the overall comprehensive program.

Engage School Staff as Advisory Team. By the time the Core Team has met with the stakeholders and collected data, there is bound to be talk in the school about future plans for suicide prevention programming. At this point, it is probably smart for the Core Team to open up involvement in the project to a larger group of staff and teachers who wish to be involved.

Practical strategy (schools): There are many different roles and responsibilities that school staff can play in a Comprehensive School-Based Suicide Prevention Program. One way to help manage the involvement of various staff is to use a checklist with the staff members listed and all the different activities in which the program will engage across the multiple columns at the top, making checkmarks in the columns in which each type of staff member might reasonably be expected to play a role (SAMHSA, 2012). For example, staff roles might include superintendent, principal, assistant principal, school nurse, school counselor(s), pupil service coordinator, special education staff, crisis response team, school psychologist, security officer, teachers, custodians, lunch staff, bus drivers, etc. The types of activities could include developing protocols for at-risk students, developing protocols for after a suicide, developing staff training, participating in staff training, developing student training, leading student training, etc. Although each school's checklist will look different, organizing the people and the projects in this way can help keep the program on track and help keep people from engaging in activities that are inappropriate for their role and function.

Although some staff will still be reluctant to engage with the topic, others will be extremely eager to consider themselves part of the advisory team. Holding a meeting with a larger group of interested staff and teachers and letting them know of the future plans can be useful.

Practical strategy (schools): As always, it is important to remember that at least some of the staff in the building will have their own personal histories with the topic. Because of their personal stories, some people will be either very willing or very unwilling to be involved. (We have found that suicide loss survivors often have one of these two extreme reactions. Rarely do we encounter someone who has a personal story with suicide—either their own thoughts or attempts or those of a student or loved one—who does not either rush to be involved or desperately wish to sit out of the process.) It is imperative that everyone in the school respect the choice of each staff and faculty member to determine their own level of involvement in the planning. It can be tempting to push or cajole another into participating in this important work, forgetting that the choice that they are making may be based on a personal story. Of course, when it comes to actually engaging in suicide prevention programming with students, we have an expectation that every staff member and teacher will participate, at a minimum, in a training on what to do to assist students. But when it comes to involvement in planning that requires efforts that are above and beyond this minimum, that is clearly at the discretion of the individual.

Engage Community Partners. Schools needs community support to help prevent suicide (Jed Foundation, 2021). In communities with existing suicide prevention coalitions, that is a great place to start. Some states have suicide prevention plans, and there is a contact person that will help school personnel navigate the appropriate partners. For a listing of state and tribal suicide prevention contacts, visit the following websites:

State contacts: http://www.sprc.org/states/all/contacts
Tribal contacts: http://www.sprc.org/grantees/listing

We also caution schools to remember that engaging in a comprehensive suicide prevention program means that there will be more students requesting services—both from the school and from the community. Having these supports in place *before the program begins* is important. In other words, encouraging students and their parents to reach out into the community for help only to find that the community is ill-prepared to respond to the additional requests can backfire. Preparing the community infrastructure for these additional referrals is important.

Practical strategy (schools): Many schools already have community resource mapping in place. In this case, we suggest that school mental health personnel extend this a bit further to know exactly what resources are available to students at risk for suicide (from all relevant cultural backgrounds and at all economic levels). Reaching out to these community supports to let them know that this intensive effort to engage the entire school in suicide prevention is important, as it warns them that they may find their resources stretched in the near future. Of course, including them in the school's suicide prevention plan, when appropriate, is even better, as integrating the existing resources into the training and education is an excellent way to help students and staff make better use of the supports that are available.

Of course, reaching out to members of specific cultural and ethnic communities that are represented within the school can be an appropriate place to find community partners for suicide prevention programming too. These community partners can help ensure that the programming that is ultimately developed is culturally responsive and effective for all students and parents (SAMHSA, 2012).

Practical strategy (schools): As always, regardless of any data or research given as evidence for the suicide prevention program, before it can be implemented within a school building, there must be clear evidence that it is culturally appropriate for the student population in the school. There is no single way to do this. Some strategies include (a) a Core Team that mirrors the cultural diversity of the student population and can represent diverse voices in the planning, implementation, and evaluation stages; (b) careful evaluation of all materials, resources, and referrals to ensure they are inclusive and respectful of all values, beliefs, cultures, and languages that are represented in the school; and (c) intentional offerings of open dialogues with members of all the student population to ensure that the material is presented in a way that is respectful to all.

The Overall Timeline for the Core Team

It may be helpful to conceptualize the work of the Core Team by visualizing this work as a timeline. Clearly, not all of the partners will be on board from the first day, and creating these different levels of partnerships will take some time. We offer the following timeline *only as a guide* to help you in your planning and to remind you that it doesn't have to happen all at once.

Sample Timeline for Core Team

Year 1: Create a Core Team.
  Core Team invites select key stakeholders to join.
  Core Team develops overall Comprehensive Suicide Prevention Program (CSPP).
  Core Team collects data on existing suicide prevention efforts at the school.
  Core Team develops and implements needs assessment.
Year 2: Add members to the Core Team from community/key stakeholders.
Expanded Core Team uses results of needs assessment to continue to refine overall CSPP.
  Expanded Core Team develops overall assessment strategy.
  Expanded Core Team works to implement beginning stages of overall CSPP.
Years 2–3: Develop a support (Advisory) Team.
  Expanded Core Team invites members to join support (Advisory) Team.
  Core and support (Advisory) Team continues to implement overall CSPP.
  Core and support (Advisory) Team collect data and use the data to make adjustments, as needed.

Step 4: Develop the Overall Strategy

Up until now, the plan has had a very general approach. Now it is time to finalize the specific strategy. It is tempting to want to include every aspect of a comprehensive program right from the start. However, we recommend a more modest approach, recognizing that schools can add components to the plan once the main aspects are ingrained in the school's culture. We try to encourage schools to consider a 5-year plan for this work, which can help this seem more manageable.

Components of a Comprehensive Approach. There are six major components to a Comprehensive School-Based Prevention Program: (a) train staff (staff education and training), (b) teach students (student education and training), (c) help parents (parent education and training), (d) engage peers (student advocates and mentors), (e) lower stigma (advocacy and anti-stigma campaigns), and (f) screen students. In the next chapter, we will discuss the specific content that should be included in the education and training. For now, we will simply give a brief outline of what they are, what decisions need to be made about if and how they should be delivered, and who needs to be involved in that decision-making process.

Train Staff. All adults in the school building (ideally, all adults who interact with students, which means the bus drivers too!) should be trained to recognize students who are at risk for suicide, to know how to respond appropriately, and to refer the student to an appropriate school staff member (e.g., school counselor, nurse, administrator) for follow-up (SAMHSA, 2012). Most in-person staff education for suicide prevention is aimed primarily for staff at the middle and high school level, although at least one available staff training program, Applied Suicide Intervention Skills Training (ASIST), has been used more broadly in K–12 schools (Shannonhouse et al., 2017).

Many of the available staff education and training programs take the form of suicide gatekeeper prevention programs. These types of programs vary in duration (from as little as an hour to as long as 2 days) and modality (in person, virtual, or blended). Although there is no clear timeline for receiving additional training, most people who study suicide prevention believe that staff will need at least some form of additional training, or at the very least, a "booster shot" at some point in the future. The timeline for this varies. The Jed Foundation (2021) recommends some follow-up training within 3–6 months after the initial gatekeeper training. Others recommend a refresher course every 2–3 years (Joshi et al., 2015). Although we agree that a shorter timeframe between trainings is ideal, we also know from experience that this might be challenging, particularly as schools start their training programs. Therefore, an additional booster training (which may be shorter than the original gatekeeper training) once per year may be an appropriate first step.

Most gatekeeper training programs share the same general common content, which includes basic information about suicide, risk factors, warning signs, and protective factors, and a strategy for how to recognize and respond to an at-risk student. Most gatekeeper training programs also include a behavioral training component (e.g., practice in how to refer the student to an appropriate staff person; Singer et al., 2019).

There are suicide prevention gatekeeper trainings available that have been rigorously tested and evaluated. Other programs might have some basic empirical support for their effectiveness without extensive data. Still other gatekeeper training programs might come from local agencies or programs. Regardless of who has authored the specific gatekeeper training program that is being considered, there are some basic considerations for the Core Team.

- The goals of the training. Although almost all gatekeeper trainings have the same core components, most also include other information or context. Does this match with the Core Team's approach?
- The cultural context of the school. The core elements of the gatekeeper training program selected must be respectful of the beliefs and language of the cultural groups represented in

the school (and be open to adaptation, as necessary and appropriate, to meet the needs of the students, staff, and teachers in the school). For additional guidance on selecting culturally appropriate suicide prevention gatekeeper trainings, see Suicide Prevention Resource Center (SPRC; 2020).

- The intended audience. Although *all* staff should be trained, it may be that some school staff require more intense training, with more advanced skills, than other staff. These are important decisions for the Core Team.
- The logistics of implementation, including the following:
  - o Length of training
  - o Depth of content
  - o Format of training
  - o Cost

In 2018, SAMHSA discontinued its National Registry of Evidence-Based Programs and Practices (NREPP) because there were no standard guidelines to determine whether the programs that were submitted were actually effective. Until a new system is in place, there is no national model to determine best practices. At the end of this chapter, we will offer a listing of some of the nationally and/or commercially available suicide prevention gatekeeper training programs. We are *not necessarily* recommending these programs, and we offer this list only as a starting place for your investigation. Until there is a national clearinghouse of evidence-based practice programs available, we can only recommend that schools use programs that offer data and evidence, in some clear format, to support their selection.

It may be helpful to classify the type of staff education you can provide into three categories. In all cases, we recommend that schools work toward the highest level of engagement, when possible, with the recognition that this may be a goal that the team works toward.

Levels of Staff Training

o Minimal
  - Crisis information At a minimum, all staff should know the crisis hotline and textline (988) as well as local resources.
  - Printed material Staff could be given printed materials in a bright red folder, for example, that has information on how to talk with a student at risk and where to turn for help, with school and local resources.
o Moderate
  - Online or video trainings, when available
o Advanced
  - In-person gatekeeper training
  - Advanced training for mental health professionals

Teach Students. Universal student education is designed to develop healthy coping skills, problem-solving skills, and a sense of social connectedness among the students. We believe that student education is important, because in spite of the high levels of depression, suicidal thoughts, ideation, and behaviors among students in all different age groups, it is clear that most children and adolescents do not receive appropriate mental health assistance. In fact, fewer than a third of adolescents who have experienced a major depressive episode within the last year received treatment (SAMHSA, 2017). The most common scenario is for suicidal young people to turn to each other for help. Adolescents, in particular, may be reluctant to seek help from adults, given their developmental needs for autonomy and independence. It is for this *very reason* that we believe it is important to go *directly to the students themselves.* Of course, we have to teach them how to get help themselves if they are feeling suicidal. We also have to help them know what to do if they believe a friend is at risk for suicide. You may recall from Chapter 1 that only 25% of teenagers say they would tell an adult if they knew a friend was contemplating suicide. When we teach students how to help their friends, we empower them to make a difference.

Importantly, student education takes place within a developmental context. Younger students (elementary age) often engage in classroom activities or classroom guidance that encourages the development of fundamental life skills. These activities might be situated within a larger module on mental health, problem-solving, decision-making, conflict resolution, loneliness prevention, and help seeking. These types of programs clearly fit within a school's resources and culture because they have an educational rather than clinical focus. They are often taught by teachers or school counselors. Often these modules focus on topics such as emotional identification or emotional expression or other types of Social and Emotional Learning (SEL). Social and emotional learning has been identified as a powerful way to build resilience and protect mental health, and there is some limited research that specifically connects these early education opportunities to reduced suicide risk in later years (Wilcox et al., 2008). The Collaborative for Advancing Social and Emotional Learning offers an extensive collection of resources for schools seeking assistance as they help develop these competencies in their students (2022).

Just because early childhood universal education does not tend to focus specifically on suicide prevention education *does not mean* that students at the elementary age cannot be suicidal. As we have noted throughout this text, childhood suicide is increasing at an alarming rate. What we are suggesting here is only that children, in general, not receive universal education that is specifically focused on suicide prevention. Adults in the elementary buildings should still receive some basic suicide prevention gatekeeper training (adapted for how suicidal behaviors might look in young children).

Older students (middle and high school) might receive universal education that is aligned more with suicide prevention. Not all schools choose to teach suicide prevention education specifically to their students, and some continue with broader life skills classes through middle and high school. However, we follow the AFSP recommendation that middle and high schools educate students on the signs and symptoms of mental health conditions, on suicide risk factors, and on how to reach out for help for themselves or their friends.

We believe that it is important to tell students, and parents, that there will be a suicide prevention training before it occurs. Some schools simply include this information in student handbooks with a general statement, such as:

> [X school] cares deeply about the health and well-being of all of our students. As part of our commitment to student safety, students in [grades x–x] will "learn about recognizing and responding to warning signs of suicide in friends, using coping skills, support systems, and seeking help for themselves and friends. This curricular content will occur in all health classes throughout the school year, not just in response to a suicide" (AFSP, 2019, p. 14).

Levels of Student Teaching

o Minimal
  • Mental health help seeking At a minimum, students in all grades should know how to seek help, who to talk to, and how to engage if they are concerned about themselves or a friend
o Moderate
  • Online modules
  • Upstream classroom strategies for elementary students
o Advanced
  • Classroom education on suicide prevention for middle and high school students

Practical strategy (schools): As we will discuss in the next chapter, one of the major takeaways from the student training is: Tell an adult if you know a friend is suicidal. We cannot stress this enough. If the message that you will tell the students is tell an adult, then the adults (all of the adults—staff, teachers, and parents) need to know what to do when a student tells them that they are worried about a friend. The adults need to be prepared for the difficult conversations that they might be having with their children about friends who are in need.

Help Parents. Parents are an important part of our school-based program. We encourage schools to have a multipronged approach to training parents. For example, we suggest that schools offer a community-based suicide prevention gatekeeper training program specifically designed for parents several times per year. Because we recognize that not all parents will (or even are able to) attend this training in person, we know it is important to get information to parents in other formats. Information via newsletters or website materials that go out to parents, particularly during high stress times (e.g., before exams or breaks or when students are receiving their college acceptance letters) can be useful.

Levels of Parental Assistance

o Minimal
   • Static information
     At a minimum, parents should have access to crisis lines, including textlines, and the local resources for suicide/mental health. This should always be available in places where parents can access information (e.g., on school website, in parent newsletters).
o Moderate
   • Online information
     It may sound "easy" to say "put information on the school's website or blogs," but the reality is that someone has to keep

that information up to date. Local resources change, information changes, and there is NOTHING worse than clicking on a link during a moment of crisis, when you need help, and the link is broken. So, if the school makes a commitment to post links on a site, then those links have to be constantly tested and updated, and that means this has to be assigned to someone as an ongoing task.

o Advanced
  - In-person education
  - Proactive messaging
    Several times per year (maybe right before academic breaks or during exams or other high stress times), messages can go out to parents, using whatever mechanism the school typically employs, with information about suicide and mental health. We encourage you NOT to create these messages, but to use one of the pre-existing credible sites (such as those on the reference page) for information to pass along to parents.

Practical strategy (schools): There is a lot of information in this chapter and a lot of preparation that needs to be done for a comprehensive school-based approach to suicide prevention. So, here is some good news. When it comes to including material in parent newsletters, this is not something that school personnel need to (or even "should") write on their own. There is high-quality information available on the web from reputable sites. Much of it is government sponsored, meaning that it can be reproduced for school use (properly cited, of course). We are happy to take at least one item, writing columns about suicide prevention, off of the Core Team's plate when it comes to the many tasks involved in suicide prevention planning!

Engage Peers. In every school, there are students who want to be involved in suicide prevention efforts. Perhaps there are student groups or organizations that are focused on mental health or students who want to do individual projects about mental health or suicide prevention advocacy for classes or in preparation for their college applications. The good news is that these students have a lot of energy and talent and they want to do the right thing. The challenging reality, however, is that these students will require some time, attention, and supervision to make sure that the projects they are doing are appropriate and align with best practices. We have so many stories (perhaps you do too!) of students who try to do the "right" thing when it comes to suicide prevention, but without appropriate adult supervision, they make decisions that are less than ideal. However, we also have great stories of students who produced the most clever videos, interactive projects, imaginative and creative ways to engage their classmates, and projects that became talking points (in the best possible way) in their schools. They found ways to engage their peers in suicide prevention in ways that we could never have imagined. Teaming up with students makes a lot of sense, but it must be done intentionally, and it takes time and commitment: This may be a terrific way to get teachers involved, with members of the Core Team simply providing consultation on content.

Levels of Peer Involvement

o Minimal

- Tap into pre-existing student groups to coordinate suicide prevention efforts.
- Ask student leaders to join a support team for suicide prevention.

o Moderate

- Create a new student group for mental health/suicide prevention.
- Participate in a pre-existing community event for suicide prevention.

o Advanced
  • Create a new event for the school to promote suicide prevention.
  • Supervise a student doing a project for suicide prevention.
  • Develop peer-to-peer campaigns within the school.
  • Train student leaders to be suicide prevention gatekeepers.

Advocacy and Anti-Stigma Campaigns. As members of the school are receiving education and training, it is likely that the entire school will want to engage in some universal approaches for advocacy and mental health promotion. There are many types of campaigns available, and we suggest starting with some of the marketing strategies available through well-known suicide prevention programs, such as AFSP or the Jed Foundation. These sites have free videos, websites, and taglines that have been properly vetted with the adolescent population. Many also have free posters, magnets, and other materials that can be used in schools or distributed to students.

Practical strategy (schools): One very promising strategy to engage the entire school in suicide prevention and to put resources directly into the hands of the people who need it most is through the use of mobile apps. These electronic resources can be used for universal prevention as well as to help struggling students who may benefit from adjuncts to selected or indicated interventions. Within mental health, apps are lauded for their multiple benefits, including anonymity, convenience, ability to provide resources inexpensively and to a large audience, and ease of access at all hours of the day and night. However, there are increasing concerns about the sheer number of mental health and suicide prevention apps that have been developed that have little to no evidence-based support for their content. Unfortunately, there are no standards in place that monitor the content of apps. There are many examples of apps that contain false or dangerous information, such as an app that informs users that Bipolar Disorder is contagious or another that states the best treatment for depression is a 'shot of whiskey' before bed (Torous, 2016).

The best strategy for using apps for suicide prevention programming and outreach within schools is to only use apps that have been vetted by a trusted organization. We offer a few examples of evidence-supported apps at the end of the chapter. When selecting apps, school personnel are reminded to stay abreast of the latest research and developments and to always make sure the content is appropriate for the culture of the school and the developmental needs of the students.

Levels of Advocacy and Outreach

o Minimal
- Post the suicide hotline/textline phone number (988) in the school building.
- Choose an existing mental health/suicide prevention campaign and join the effort in your school.

o Moderate
- Reach out to local or national resources for some swag (e.g., pens, laptop stickers, posters) to share with students.

o Advanced
- Create your own campaign. Use the creativity of your students, incorporate the concepts of suicide prevention/ help seeking and your school logo or mascot, and make school-specific logo and swag. Personalizing these advocacy messages really sends home the message that your school cares.

Practical strategy (schools): We encourage schools to make full use of the materials and information available from local, state, and national suicide prevention organizations. For example, local chapters will often provide free materials for distribution at school events. Remember, the goal of all of this is to get material into the hands of students. We vividly remember conducting a training of school counselors at a site where we had conducted a training a few years previously. At the first training, we recommended that the participants contact a national organization for free magnets with the suicide prevention hotline number and post them in the bathrooms, noting that adolescents (particularly boys) are more likely to call the hotline than to talk with an adult in person, and bathrooms are a "safe" place for them to make note of the hotline number. At our subsequent training, a participant raised their hand and said, "I did what you told me, and I got those free magnets, and I put them in the bathrooms at our school, and the kids stole them—so I won't do that anymore." We were astounded. Of course, if the students took the free magnets with the hotline number, our response was, then please get some more free magnets and put them in the bathroom. Clearly the students want the information. After all, the point of advocacy and anti-stigma campaigns is to get information and resources in the hands of students.

Screen Students. Screening for suicide and related mental health conditions can be an important component of a school-based comprehensive program. Screening can be universal or with students who are known to be at risk (Singer et al., 2019). Generally, screening involves two steps: the actual screening process and a follow-up individual interview to determine whether more intensive intervention is warranted (Juhnke et al., 2011). Although universal screening programs are ideal to identify students who may be suicidal *before* they exhibit signs of suicide, we recognize that there are logistical issues that must be in place before this type of screening program can begin. Some of the questions that the Core Team will want to consider include:

- Who will be screened? Is this the entire school (universal), only a particular grade, or only students who are already known to be at risk (indicated). If it is only indicated students, how will they be identified?
- What screening instrument will be used? Again, at the end of this chapter, we will provide some suggestions, but without

a best practices registry available, there are no clear answers. Whatever instrument is selected should have sound psychometric properties and be appropriate for the student population (including being developmentally and culturally appropriate).

- What staffing is required to complete the screening and the follow-up face-to-face interviews?
- What referrals are available to the students who screen positive?
- How will the screening program be monitored to ensure that proper protocols are being followed?
- How will informed consent be obtained from parents/ guardians?
- How will the screening program be funded?

We know from first-hand experience that a large-scale screening program in K–12 can be challenging. It can also save lives. In our work, we helped develop Ohio's Adolescent Mental Health Screening Program, which was funded through SAMHSA to screen middle and high school students in Ohio. Over the course of 3 years, nearly 14,000 students were screened using Columbia's TeenScreen. Here is some of what we learned:

- Parental consent is an important question. In our work, we decided to use active parental consent, meaning students had to return a signed permission slip. With active consent, we had a 33% participation rate. Others believe that passive consent (parents have to opt out) is sufficient (e.g., Scott et al., 2009). With passive consent, Scott and colleagues achieved double the consent rate, about 67%. However, given the controversial nature of screening, we chose active consent, even though it meant a lower participation rate. What you choose has a lot to do with the culture of your school and your local regulations and laws. Whether using active or passive parental consent, all screening programs also require student assent. In other words, for the program to effectively screen students, the students themselves must agree to participate.

- Every student must be given the option to talk with someone. Whether the student has a "positive" screen or not, after the screening, each student should be given the opportunity to speak with a mental health professional, if they desire, and be given information about referrals and resources.

- Arranging for individual interviews is time consuming and represented the most expensive part of our process. Our protocol included a 30-minute interview with a mental health professional for each student who had a positive screen. The goal of this interview was not to make a clinical diagnosis, but to determine if the student could benefit from follow-up assessment or intervention (or to determine if an emergency referral was necessary). Approximately 24% of students scored positive on the screen (about 3,300 students) and required a follow-up interview. This is consistent with most of the screening instruments.

- Not everyone who scores positive on the screening instruments is suicidal or even has a mental health problem. In fact, one of the criticisms of all of the suicide and mental health screening instruments is that they have a high rate of false positives. That is, they tend to "catch" students who are in distress for a variety of reasons, not all of which are related to mental health or suicide. Students might be upset about schoolwork or career choices, for example, and in these instances require assistance from tutors or teachers or the school counselor. In our work, about 59% of the students who received the 30-minute follow-up clinical interviews required a referral to a mental health professional for a more intensive assessment. When this occurred, parents were encouraged to meet with school personnel regarding the screening results and were given a follow-up appointment with a mental health professional for a more intensive assessment and necessary interventions.

- In our program, even when parents gave active permission for the screening, students screened positive, and mental health professionals met with the students and confirmed the results of the screening, not all parents followed through with the follow-up appointments. In fact, even when we were able to set up and *pay for* the referrals for the students who had the positive screens, only about half of the parents followed through on these appointments. This underscores the *stigma* that still exists for mental health and suicide.

We know that not every school will be part of a large federally funded project to offer suicide and mental health screening to their students. In fact, we recognize that most schools *will not* have this luxury. Nevertheless, we also know that there is a very real, very tangible benefit to students if schools can make this happen for their students. So, we encourage schools to not simply dismiss the idea. Perhaps there is something that your school can do? This might not be part of a school's first stage of a Comprehensive School-Based Suicide Prevention Program, but we encourage you to keep it in mind as you develop your long-term strategy.

Step 5: Implement an Evaluation Plan

As with every program, evaluation is both the first and the last component. Measuring the effectiveness of each component of the program, as well as the overall program, allows for important changes and updates to occur. For example, pre-post questionnaires of teachers and staff on knowledge and skills (confidence and competence) as well as willingness to engage if they believe a student is at risk for suicide are important measures of the staff education component. Other evaluation strategies might include measuring the number of students who have been referred to the school counselor by staff and teachers, or the number of referrals that have been made to outside agencies. Customizing the specific evaluation components to reflect the needs of the school, based on specific variables such as racial diversity, school size, or poverty effects, might provide a context to the data that can be particularly helpful as the Core Team tries to make sense of the data they are reviewing (Granello & Zyromski, 2019). Finally, we will remind you again that we specifically caution *against* any evaluation plan using suicide behaviors (e.g., completed suicides, hospitalizations) as part of the outcome measures. In spite of the best programming efforts, suicide is a complex phenomenon that is affected by many variables within a child's life, many of which are beyond the scope of the school. Linking evaluation to outcomes that are reasonably within the control of the program is a *far better* choice.

Conclusion

Schools have an important role to play in suicide prevention. Universal prevention models are based on a public health approach. They help limit stigma, increase help seeking, and promote strategies to reach out to those at risk. The most commonly used universal approaches are staff education and gatekeeper training, student education, parent education, peer-to-peer engagement, anti-stigma campaigns, and school-based mental health screening. Although the research on these types of programming varies significantly, all of these types of interventions have initial empirical support as methods to reduce suicide risk in schools.

Suicide Gatekeeper Training (Primarily for Staff Education)

- **Question, Persuade, Refer (QPR)**
  o Staff education
  o 90 minutes

- Applied Suicide Intervention Skills Training (ASIST)
  - o Staff education
  - o 14 hours
- Kognito At-Risk for High School and Middle School Educators
  - o Staff education
  - o Online modules

Universal Student Education Programs

- Good Behavior Game (GBG)
  - o First and second grade
  - o Student education program
- Promoting Alternative Thinking Strategies (PATHS)
  - o Pre-K, elementary, and middle school
  - o Student education program
- Online Suicide Prevention for High School Students
  - The state of Michigan, in coordination with Blue Cross/Blue Shield, has developed a free online professional development course for high school students. This training has not been empirically validated. It is available at https://michiganvirtual.org/adolescent-suicide-prevention/.
- Signs of Suicide (SOS)
  - o Middle and high school
  - o Student education and screening
- Sources of Strength (SOS)
  - o Middle and high school
  - o Student education
- American Indian Life Skills Development Curriculum (AILSD)
  - o High school
  - o Student education

- Linking Education and Awareness of Depression and Suicide (LEADS)
  o High school
  o Student education
- Lifelines Curriculum
  o Middle and high school
  o Student education

Note: All programs listed here demonstrated at least "promising" levels of effectiveness based on their initial reviews with SAMHSA's National Registry of Evidence-Based Programs and Practices (NREPP). However, that registry was discontinued in 2018 and has not been replaced. Therefore, without a national registry of evidence-based practice, these programs are <u>not</u> offered as recommendations, only as available models. School personnel are <u>strongly encouraged</u> to review the existing data and evidence, as well as the relevance of any program they wish to adopt with the students in their school, before they consider the use of any specific program.

Mobile Apps

Apps for Universal Suicide Prevention Programming

- A Friend Asks (Jason Foundation) A free app designed to teach users how to recognize the signs that someone close to them may be thinking about suicide, and how to reach out to them proactively.
- Suicide Safe (SAMHSA) Provides tips and real time "what to do" action steps. It is also used by mental health providers and therefore, includes suicide assessment and triage information
- You are Important (It Gets Better) This app is specifically designed for LGB youth and focuses on the message, You Are Important.

Apps for Selective/Indicated Interventions

My3 (California Suicide Prevention Campaign and Suicide Prevention Resource Center) This app connects potentially suicidal people to their support system, their safety plans, and to the hotline.

This list is by no means exhaustive and is intended only as a starting place. Further, although mobile apps can be useful, one study (Martinengo et al., 2019) found that of 46 widely available suicide prevention apps, only one in ten contained the minimum necessary information to be useful (for example, only 51% of the apps studied had any educational content). Therefore, caution must be taken when recommending these apps to students and others in the school. Always use reputable sites for these apps, keep abreast of the latest changes and developments in the field, and download and test the apps first to make sure they are appropriate for your school.

References

American Foundation for Suicide Prevention. (2019). *Model school district policy on suicide prevention.*

Collaborative for Advancing Social and Emotional Learning (CASEL). (2022). *CASAL guide to schoolwide SEL.* Available from: https://casel.org/

Gordon, R. (1987). An operational classification of disease prevention. In: J. A. Steinberg, editor; and M. M. Silverman, Eds. Preventing Mental Disorders. Rockville, MD: Department of Health and Human Services; 20–26.

Gould, M. S., Marracco, F. A., Kleinman, M., Thomas, J. G., Mostkoff, K., Cote, J., & Davies, M. (2005). Evaluating iatrogenic risk of youth suicide screening programs: A randomized controlled trial. *Journal of the American Medical Association, 293*(13), 1635–1643.

Granello, P. F., & Zyromski, B. (2019). Developing a comprehensive school suicide prevention program. *Professional School Counseling, 22*(1), 1–11. doi:10.1177/2156759X18808128

Jed Foundation. (2021). *A comprehensive approach to mental health promotion and suicide prevention for high schools.* http://www.jedfoundation.org

Joshi, S. V., Ojakian, M., Lenoir, L., Hartley, S., & Weitz, E. (2015). *Comprehensive suicide toolkit for schools.* Palo Alto Unified School District.

Juhnke, G. A., Granello, D. H., & Granello, P. F. (2011). *Suicide, self-injury, and violence in the schools: Assessment, prevention, and intervention strategies*. Wiley.

Katz, C., Bolton, S-L., Katz, L. Y., Isaak, C., Tilston-Jones, T., Sareen, J., & Swampy Cree Suicide Prevention Teams. (2013). A systematic review of school-based suicide prevention programs. *Depression and Anxiety, 30*, 1030–1045.

Martinengo, L., Van Galen, L, Lum, E., Kowalski, M., Subramaniam, M., & Car, J. (2019). Suicide prevention and depression apps' suicide risk assessment and management: A systematic assessment of adherence to clinical guidelines. *BMC Medication, 17*(1), 231. doi: 10.1186/s12916-019-1461-z

Scott, M. A., Wilcox, H. C., Schonfeld, I. S., Davies, M., Hicks, R. C., Turner, J. B., & Shaffer, D. (2009). School-based screening to identify at-risk students not already known to school professionals: The Columbia Suicide Screen. *American Journal of Public Health, 99*, 224–339.

Shannonhouse, L., Lin, Y. W. D., Shaw, K., & Porter, M. (2017). Suicide intervention training for K-12 schools: A quasi-experimental study on ASIST. *Journal of Counseling and Development, 99*, 3–13. doi:10-1002/jcad.12112

Singer, J. B., Erbacher, T. A., & Rosen, P. (2019). School-based suicide prevention: A framework for evidence-based practice. *School Mental Health, 11*, 54–71. doi:10.1007/s12310-018-9245-8

Smith-Millman, M. K., & Flaspohler, P. D. (2019). School-based suicide prevention laws in action: A nationwide investigation of principals' knowledge of and adherence to state school-based suicide prevention laws. *School Mental Health, 11*, 321–334.

Substance Abuse and Mental Health Services Administration. (2012). *Policies and protocols addressing the needs of youths who have attempted or are considering suicide*. https://sprc.org/sites/default/files/migrate/library/LLWG_Policies%20and%20Protocols_2012.pdf

Substance Abuse and Mental Health Services Administration. (2017). *National Survey on Drug Use and Health*. https://nsduhweb.rti.org/

Suicide Prevention Resource Center. (2020). *Guidance for culturally adapting gatekeeper trainings*. https://www.sprc.org/sites/default/files/Guidance%20for%20Culturally%20Adapting%20Gatekeeper%20Trainings.pdf

Torous, J. (2016). How mental health apps are regulated—or are they? *Psychiatric Times. https://www.psychiatrictimes.com/view/how-mental-health-apps-are-regulatedor-are-they*

U.S. Department of Health and Human Services (HHS) Office of the Surgeon General and National Action Alliance for Suicide Prevention. (2012, September). *2012 National strategy for suicide prevention: Goals and objectives for action*. https://pubmed.ncbi.nlm.nih.gov/23136686/

Walrath, C., Garraza, L. G., Reid, H., Goldston, D. B., & McKeon, R. (2015). Impact of the Garrett Lee Smith youth suicide prevention program on suicide mortality. *American Journal of Public Health, 105*, 986–993. doi:10.2105/AJPH.2014.302496

Washington County Department of Public Health & Environment. (2001). *Adolescent depression and suicide opinion survey.* http://www.co.washing ton.mn.us/client_files/documents/FHL-teensurv.pdf

Wilcox, H. C., Kellam, S. G., Brown, C. H., Poduska, J., Ialongo, N. S., Wang, W., & Anthony, J. C. (2008). The impact of two universal randomized first and second grade classroom interventions on young adult suicide ideation and attempt. *Drug and Alcohol Dependence, 95*(Suppl. 1), S60–S73. doi:10.1016/j.drugalcdep.2008.01.005

7

School-Based Suicide Prevention Programming

The "Nuts and Bolts" of Education and Training

In this chapter, we turn our attention to action, implementation, and education. Once the groundwork has been laid, the data has been collected, the framework has been established, the protocols are in place, and the school is ready, the training can begin. In the following sections, we will give you the current strategies, based on the research, for training teachers, students, and parents in suicide prevention. We will also share with you our approach for establishing a comprehensive school-based training and the specific strategy that we use and recommend. We will share reactions and feedback from those we have trained and very specific ideas and suggestions you might want to try. We want to be clear, however, that at the current moment, *there is no national evidence-based best practice strategy* for suicide prevention programming in the schools. All we can offer is the current thinking, supported by research whenever possible, and results from our own work, which is grounded in that research as well as supported by our own research and data. In our own work, we collect data on every training, and we have a lot of evidence that the overall strategy that we use is effective. However, we also know that as individual schools apply any of these programs, as we have repeatedly said, it is important to adapt everything that is written here to the needs of the students in the school and to collect data to determine the program's effectiveness for the students, staff, teachers, and parents involved.

Suicide and Self-Injury in Schools. Darcy Haag Granello, Paul F. Granello, Gerald A. Juhnke,
Oxford University Press. © Oxford University Press 2023. DOI: 10.1093/oso/9780190059842.003.0007

Implementing the Plan: Suicide Prevention Programming

The goal of universal suicide prevention programming is to give everyone in the building at least some knowledge, awareness, and skills to be an effective part of the comprehensive approach. However, as we cautioned in the last chapter, an effective plan is a clear and methodical one that is intentional about training each group appropriately, and in the right order. Toward that end, in this section, we will give specific recommendations for how each of these major groups should receive their training.

Staff Training

In most schools, the first group to receive any training will be the staff. We have found that this typically works best when it occurs before the start of the academic year, although we also have done these trainings during other in-service days throughout the year, if that works better with staff calendars.

Training the Mental Health Professionals. It is possible, and in fact probable, that different staff will require different levels of training with varying levels of intensity and focus. For example, the Core Team might determine that all of the staff in the school who are mental health professionals or administrators who interact with potentially suicidal students should first receive a more advanced clinical training in suicide assessment and intervention. This makes sense, since typically the purpose of the other trainings in the school is to learn how to refer a potentially suicidal student to the appropriate school professional for more advanced assessment and care. That clearly means that there is a tier of individuals at the school who must have advanced training. We recognize that this type of training perhaps fits more closely with selected intervention and assessment, which we will discuss in the next two chapters.

However, we mention it here because it is not okay to train the rest of the school in a broad-based universal intervention approach to suicide prevention until at least some members of the school team have received this more advanced training and education.

It is not wise to assume that all school mental health professionals receive this advanced training in suicide assessment and intervention during their graduate education. In fact, most do not. Across all the helping professions, there are large and well-documented gaps in graduate education related to suicide assessment and intervention. For example, in national studies, only about 21% of social workers, 40% of school psychologists, and 70% of school counselors had *any training* during their graduate programs in any aspect of suicide (Schmidt, 2016). Even among those who had been trained during their graduate programs, most school-based mental health professionals have significant concerns about their ability to recognize a student at risk for suicide, even after years on the job (National Action Alliance for Suicide Prevention, 2014).

The good news is that after receiving appropriate training, school-based mental health professionals have appropriate levels of confidence to conduct risk assessments of students and to engage in appropriate ongoing management of students (Singer & Slovak, 2011; Schmidt, 2016). Importantly, this practitioner-level training appears to be an important step in keeping some school-based mental health professionals from becoming *overconfident* and relying solely on their informal impressions of the student, rather than on more formal, structured assessment interviews, which provide better outcomes (Schmidt, 2016). Bringing all staff who require this advanced training up to the same level, using the same assessments and intervention protocols, is an important first step. We will provide further information on suicide risk assessment in the next chapter.

It is important to mention here (and we will discuss this more thoroughly in the next chapter) that the role of school mental health professionals is typically *not* to complete comprehensive suicide risk assessments. In fact, most of the professional associations (e.g., American School Counselor Association, National Association of School Psychologists) specifically caution against definitive suicide risk assessment by school professionals. However, someone in the school (and this is often the school counselor, school psychologist, or school nurse) must make a determination if a call should be made to a parent and a student requires a referral to an outside source for a risk assessment, and this is the type of risk assessment training to which we are referring.

> *Practical strategy (schools): We know that it can be difficult to find the appropriate training on this type of suicide risk assessment for school staff. When possible, we recommend that school mental health professionals reach out to local universities to determine if there is someone who might assist with this training (or to recommend qualified individuals who are available to assist).*

Training the Staff. The rest of the staff will all need to be trained to know how to recognize a student who might be at risk and to intervene to get that student to the appropriate person to conduct the appropriate risk assessment. As a reminder, *all school staff* ideally means *everyone who interacts with students:* teachers, coaches, clerical staff, lunchroom personnel, custodial staff, bus drivers—the list goes on and on. What we know from experience (and many people in school buildings reinforce this message) is that some of the students who are at highest risk often have close relationships with the support staff, and it is essential that these staff also have this important knowledge and skill. At the university where we work, for example, we make extra efforts to train our housekeeping staff, because they are often among the first people to recognize when students change their habits about leaving their dorm rooms. In K–12 buildings, there are staff who also are aware of these changes to students' normal routines. One of us works closely with a server in a middle school cafeteria. She has come to know all of the students' meal choices and preferences, and the students know her by name and confide in her. She isn't a full-time staff person, and she isn't normally part of the school's in-service education. Yet when something changes in the school or with a student, she is often the first to know. She is a prime example of *why* we train everyone, not just the teachers and administrators, in suicide prevention.

Whenever possible, we try to train all the staff during the same week or month, so that all staff receive this training at approximately the same time. This is helpful, because it means that we can move forward with student education, knowing that every adult in the school is prepared to answer student questions, at least minimally, and can refer students to appropriate resources.

Typically, the type of training that is done with staff is called suicide prevention gatekeeper training. These gatekeeper trainings are done in relatively small groups of 25–30 people at a time. Certainly, some models allow for groups that are a bit larger—maybe even up to 50 people, but often not much larger than that. Our own research conducted using focus groups of gatekeeper training participants reinforces the need for smaller groups, which is consistently mentioned by those who have been trained as important to their own learning. This is difficult material for many people, and smaller groups allow for more interaction. It also means that the group leader can scan the group, watch the reactions of the group members, and check to make sure all is well. Finally, because gatekeeper training has a behavioral component, smaller groups allow for skill development and feedback.

The specific model that a school uses will depend on the logistics of the suicide prevention gatekeeper training that the core team selects. We use a model that is 90 minutes long. Other models use longer timeframes (some use a shorter time block, although we have not encountered any that is shorter than 60 minutes). We know of only one, Kognito (Albright et al., 2016), that uses an entirely virtual format.

Practical strategy (schools): Whenever a school system develops a strategy designed to train all staff, including those in support roles, we like to send a simple yet important cautionary reminder. Not all staff in these support roles have literacy skills, and not all staff will necessarily be able to participate if the material is written, even if it is written in the participant's native language. Staff who work in roles that typically do not require them to engage in classroom education, with PowerPoint slides and handouts, do not necessarily learn this way. Learn from our humbling experience here. Handing out materials or projecting slides with information to groups that do not have basic literacy is a quick way to disenfranchise the very group you are trying to bring along as your allies. It is useful to work with representatives of these groups in advance to make sure that the materials are presented in a format and learning style that is best for their needs.

Regardless of the format, the time allowed, and the learning styles of the participants, the content of the staff training, in general, follows the same suicide prevention gatekeeper training approach. There is a lot of research on gatekeeper training programs within educational systems, and overall evidence shows that this type of training of staff holds promise as part of an overall strategy to combat suicide (Isaac et al., 2009). In addition, the available research demonstrates that there are specific areas where gatekeeper training has the most impact. These include the ability of this type of training to change knowledge, beliefs, attitudes, self-efficacy, and skills (Yonemoto et al., 2019). That means that staff training should address these areas, at a minimum. We recommend the following strategy to address these core areas:

- Basic material about suicide (knowledge)
  o Brief information on myths, overviews, basic statistics
- Risk factors, warning signs, and protective factors (knowledge)
  o Emphasis on specific risk factors for student population within school

o Recognition of specific risks among cultural groups or high-risk students
- Many suicides can be prevented (beliefs)
o The role of stigma, other barriers to help seeking
- The school has a role to play in suicide prevention (attitudes)
o How a school-wide culture of care can promote help seeking
- The person being trained has a role to play in suicide prevention (attitudes)
o Each person must feel competent, confident, and willing to intervene.
- A behavioral strategy or approach for responding (skills)
o It might be helpful to develop a simple mnemonic or strategy to remind each staff member or teacher to ASK about suicide and REFER the student to the appropriate school mental health professional.
- All of the available research (Substance Abuse Mental Health Services Administration [SAMHSA], 2012) and decades of our own experience and research conducting gatekeeper training with more than 30,000 participants tell us that the opportunity to practice these difficult conversations with students is one of the most important parts of suicide gatekeeper training. Practice role plays are consistently identified by participants as essential to their learning.
- Practice with the behavioral strategy (self-efficacy)
o Role plays or small group practice
o Most staff and teachers will need time and practice, and acknowledgment that these are very difficult and uncomfortable conversations. However, with training, they will also need support and validation that they *can* engage with students appropriately and help prevent suicide.

Practical strategy (schools): We encourage gatekeepers to be "gently persistent" when they engage with troubled students. That is, if the gatekeeper approaches a student and asks if they are okay or would like to talk, the gatekeeper should not accept the first "no" or "I'm fine"—but instead gently continue the conversation and encourage the student to seek help. That is because when others ask how they are, most people will respond with "I'm fine" the first time the question is asked. The reality is, getting at the real answer might take a bit more probing. Many school staff find it difficult to encourage discussion without feeling overly intrusive. This is why role playing and other opportunities for practice are such essential components for gatekeeper training.

At the conclusion of the gatekeeper training, we make an effort to certify everyone. We provide each participant with a printed certificate that has the participant's name already filled in (not a blank one that they fill in, but one that already has their name and that is individually signed by the right people too!). Some schools also provide participants with a pin that they can add to the lanyard of their nametag or some other indication that they have been through the training. We believe that these extra efforts are important. We are trying to raise the self-efficacy of those who have been trained. We want them to take the training seriously—and to believe that they are now capable of *doing something different.* Ending the training with a hard copy of a signed certificate that *already has their name on it* and that they come to the front of the room to receive from the trainer, who looks them in the eye and says congratulations, means more than a blank certificate that they receive electronically and fill in. We know this. They *feel* different. It is important.

We encourage everyone who has received a certificate of training to post it publicly (school offices, classrooms, front of the bus, etc.). We have found that those who wish to be proactive and communicate to students that they are approachable are quick to put up their certificates. Thus, it is important that the certificate be written in a way that communicates to students that this adult is willing to engage in difficult discussions. A certificate that reads "This Certifies That Mr/s. XX Has Completed a Suicide Prevention Training" doesn't send the complete message. In our experience, having a small group of faculty and administrators (and perhaps students) develop a certificate that is meaningful to students within the culture of that school is much more appropriate. For example, "XX Is a Certified Suicide Prevention Gatekeeper [date] and Is Part of XX School's Culture of Care"—or "XX is trained and ready to help if you or a friend is thinking about suicide . . ." whatever words make sense for your school building.

> *Practical strategy (schools): Although all staff must have minimum competencies in suicide prevention, we know that not all school staff feel equally comfortable in this role. Of course, students should be able to approach any adult in the school with their concerns. Nevertheless, there are some people who will really respond to the training and will want to communicate to students that they are available and willing to help. We have seen some school staff and teachers go "above and beyond" and create an extra layer—some sign that they post on their doors or in their classrooms or offices that signals to the students that they are <u>very open</u> to the conversation. Something simple works best. We have seen slogans such as "You Can Talk to Me" or "I Am Here to Help" or even "I Specialize in Difficult Conversations." Another school simply asked teachers and staff to post blue dots (recognizing that blue dots could be put on laptops, coffee cups, etc.). You can do whatever works best in your building. Then, when the students go through their training, they can be encouraged to talk with any adult in the school building, or they can seek out adults who have these signs posted, knowing that these are adults who might be particularly easy to talk to. For students who are struggling to open up to the school counselor, this could feel like a safe pathway in.*

Student Training

In the absence of accurate information, teenagers will look for answers wherever they can find them. They will ask their friends, attempt to make up answers for themselves, or use the Internet, where suicide information is easily accessible but of highly unpredictable quality. Of course, as we discussed in Chapter 4, they will also use social media to discuss their own, and others' suicidal thoughts and behaviors. Again, the quality of the information on these social media platforms is highly variable, ranging from posts that encourage help seeking to posts and pages that teach clear methods for suicide completion or advice on how to write a suicide note.

We are strong advocates for developmentally appropriate student education and training in suicide prevention. We believe that it is important for adults to impose ourselves into these important dialogues—to give students accurate information, to help lower the stigma for help seeking, and to teach them how to seek appropriate help. We are laying the foundation for a lifetime of healthy coping, and it is important to start early.

Elementary Education on Mental Health.   Younger students, such as those in pre-K and the elementary grades, benefit most from classroom guidance activities that lay the foundation for healthy behaviors, rather than from specific discussions on suicide risk and warning signs. Education that focuses on protective factors, such as coping skills, emotion regulation strategies, and how to reach out to caring adults, can be useful to decrease the likelihood of the development of risk factors that are associated with later suicidal behavior. Programs that help children feel connected to the school, to family, and to the community and provide opportunities to participate and make contributions also are important in developing strong protective factors.

Some schools may use existing programs. The PAX Good Behavior Game is for first and second graders. It has been shown to help decrease the development of later suicide ideation and attempt (Wilcox et al., 2008). The Promoting Alternative Thinking Strategies (PATHS; Sheftall et al., 2020) has options for pre-K, elementary, and middle school students and helps decrease emotional dysregulation, a known risk factor for suicide.

Although both of these programs show promise, we recognize that not all schools will choose to use one of these models, either because of lack of access or because they have other programs in place to address the development of social and emotional learning among their youngest students. As long as these programs address these important skills, we cannot say that the current models should be abandoned. We simply know that the ability to accurately identify and appropriately express emotions is one of the most important skills that young children can learn. In pre-K and elementary schools where pre-existing programming is not available, we suggest the PBS Kids *Mister Rogers* spinoff, *Daniel Tiger's Neighborhood*, which teaches children emotional identification and expression by providing a model for emotional regulation. There are, of course, many other games and activities that help children with this important life skill. The important thing is to provide ample opportunities to explore emotions in a safe environment and to learn how to express and manage emotions.

Regardless of the quality of this education, it will not prevent all suicidal behaviors in children. Although suicide among elementary age children remains relatively rare, it is on the rise. Supportive school environments and education that helps children develop important life skills may help, but the reality is that many children with significant mental health concerns go undetected within elementary schools. Further, when very young children die by suicide, it is often not the result of psychopathology, but because of relationship problems with family and friends (Sheftall et al., 2016). This is different from suicide among adolescents, where relationship conflicts are often with boyfriends and girlfriends. For very young children, the most common precipitating factor before a suicide is interpersonal conflict with friends and family. That means that school staff and teachers who interact with children on a daily basis need to recognize that when they are in the midst of relationship turmoil and do not have the skills to navigate this conflict, they need help. In addition to teaching children interpersonal conflict resolution, positive emotional skill development, and emotional regulation, staff and teachers must be trained to step in and assist by helping to negotiate conflict, when necessary. We also believe that when elementary staff receive their suicide gatekeeper training, they need to be taught how risk factors and warning signs might look different for young children.

> *Practical strategy (schools): There is exciting new research that demonstrates that building resilience in elementary-aged children results in both short-term and long-term gains across multiple domains, including reducing anxiety, depressive symptoms, and general psychological distress. It also appears that once learned, re-silience helps limit both internalizing and externalizing symptoms. Universal resilience education appears to be an approach that holds more promise for elementary-aged students than for adolescents. Although many different types of programs fall into this category, in general, the focus is on building and maintaining positive mental health, particularly in the midst of, or following, adversity. School-based resiliency development approaches can take a variety of formats, including curriculum-based lessons and/or broader-based school-wide strategies (Dray et al., 2017).*

Middle and High School Student Education on Suicide.   In grades 7–12, classroom activities should include more direct education in suicide, depression, and mental health. These sessions usually consist of several class periods, often included in the health curriculum. These types of classroom activities represent a valuable method of communicating to a large number of students without extensive staff time. The content of a suicide prevention classroom activity can include information about suicide risk factors and warning signs, the dispelling of suicide myths, how to recognize warning signs in others, where to go for resources to help, and how to respond to a troubled friend. An important focus of classroom activities for adolescents is to lessen the stigma about help seeking and to stress the importance of talking to a trusted adult if they are concerned about a fellow student. Essentially, **get help for yourself, and get help for a friend.**

Further, students should be helped to understand that suicidal thoughts and feelings may be part of a mental illness, such as depression or bipolar disorder. We have found that it is important to help adolescents understand that mental illness can and should be treated. It is not a sign of character weakness. Finally, adolescents need to understand that feeling sad and even fleeting thoughts of suicide are normal (and it doesn't mean they are "crazy" to think about suicide)—*but acting on those suicidal thoughts is not okay.* In other words, normalize that many people feel frustrated and overwhelmed, but that doesn't mean they kill themselves.

In general, classroom activities are intended to destigmatize seeking adult help. Adolescents may have a misplaced sense of loyalty to their friends, believing that keeping a friend's suicidal intent secret is the "right" thing to do. In one of our trainings with a group of high school boys, we reinforced the importance of telling an adult if they believed a friend was suicidal. Midway through the training, a student raised his hand and said, "I think I understand what you are telling us. *It's better to lose a friendship than to lose a friend.*" We have been repeating that "slogan" in our trainings ever since.

Suicide education should take care to emphasize the complexity of suicide. There are no easy answers to understanding suicide, and simplistic explanations can send the wrong message to students, that suicide is somehow a "solution" to life's problems. Education programs also must help students understand that although it is important for them to reach out and tell an adult if they think a friend is suicidal, *they are not responsible for keeping anyone else alive and should never be put in a position of feeling responsible for another's safety.* Many students will know someone who has completed suicide or made an attempt, and they must not be made to feel responsible for that person's decision. Always include a list of crisis intervention resources and hotline numbers in every training (including textline information). This is particularly important for males, as boys may be more likely to reach out to a crisis line than to an individual in person. Make sure someone is available to talk with students individually after the training if they need to process the material with an adult. Finally, there are specific curricular choices that are important to avoid, as research demonstrates that they may increase suicide risk. These are:

Never talk about suicide as a reaction to stress, as this can inadvertently normalize suicide (Doan et al., 2012).

Never talk about suicide as a way to end pain (as in "he killed himself because he was in so much pain").

Avoid presentations (in person or via media) of other young people who have made a suicide attempt or media depictions of suicidal behaviors, in case students overidentify with the person or model the behavior. Rather, focus on how people reached out and got help.

There are several available suicide education programs for students, which we discussed in the previous chapter. The most well researched is Signs of Suicide (SOS; Aseltine et al., 2007). Others, such as Linking Education and Awareness of Depression and Suicide (LEADS; SAVE.org, 2021) and the Lifelines Prevention Curriculum (Hazelden, 2018), also have some evidence of effectiveness. The Sources of Strength program (SOS, Wyman et al., 2010) focuses more on the development of protective factors and on health promotion than specifically on suicide prevention education. As we noted previously, all of the research on suicide prevention programming in schools is currently under review by SAMHSA.

We have a general approach to training high school students that is easily and quickly adapted to the specific needs of a school or age group. First, universal approaches emphasize the importance of training all students. Therefore, finding a class or time that includes all students is essential. However, suicide education training *should never occur* within the context of a large school assembly. Students need time and space to process these difficult topics, and smaller classroom settings are much more appropriate. Research is clear that large or auditorium-based training is *never a good idea* (Juhnke et al., 2011).

We recommend training an entire grade level during the course of a week-long effort. For example, a school might decide to train all ninth graders in health class through a series of education sessions. In general, we use a mix of approaches within the education session, relying on discussion, media, and role play. We also present information about suicide risk within the broader context of mental health.

We do not participate in "one shot" trainings. A single session does not allow students time to reflect and ask questions. If they are left with concerns or unanswered questions, they do not have time for follow-up. We have found that a suicide prevention education program, situated within the context of a health class or other curriculum that includes discussion of mental health, works best. Our typical trainings are Monday/Wednesday or Tuesday/Thursday. This two-shot approach allows students to go home with some information after the first day, spend some time thinking about what they have learned, and get any questions answered on the second day. It also prevents us from doing education in the topic on Friday and sending students home to wait over the weekend to have their questions answered.

Practical strategy (schools): We discussed this specific strategy in Chapter 3, but it is worth repeating here as you develop your curriculum for student education. Differentiating between depression and sadness is essential, and student education on suicide is an ideal time to help students understand the difference. Because many people use the words "depressed" and "sad" interchangeably, it can be confusing for students (and adults, too). Clinical depression is not the same thing as sadness. Depression is a major medical illness that adversely affects more than just mood. It also affects how people think, act, feel, and manage their lives. Helping the students (and adults) we train differentiate between depression and sadness isa critical component of all of our education and training.

Finally, we are clear that the suicide prevention education curriculum is not intended to address suicidal feelings or behaviors directly. Rather, these sessions emphasize help-seeking skills and resources and are primarily designed for students who come into contact with distressed peers. We recognize that there will be students in the room who are in distress themselves, and we are careful to provide resources and referrals for students, but we do not engage in counseling during the training.

We offer the following general outline for a suicide prevention education curriculum. There are many ways that schools can provide this education to their students, and we are not suggesting that this is the only approach. Nevertheless, it is an approach that has worked well for us.

Day 1 (1 hour):

- Introduce the topic.
- Discuss suicide myths, risk factors, and warning signs. (Help students make sense of some of the myths they have heard and learn how to recognize risk in themselves and others. Including information about stigma is important.)
- Provide a very brief presentation of statistics and general information for their age group. (This can help young people recognize that they are not alone.)

- Discuss protective factors. (Help students recognize that there are things that they can do. Thinking about suicide does not *inevitably* lead to suicide behaviors. This is important. There is some emerging evidence that some students are starting to think that because they are hearing so much about suicide, this is just the ultimate path that will happen to at least some of their classmates—maybe to them. Instilling hope early in the talk means that they recognize that there is another path.)
- Role play: What is the difference between feeling sad and feeling depressed? (Sad is a feeling that all of us experience. Depression is a clinical diagnosis and requires more intensive assistance. When teens know the difference, they start to recognize why depression isn't something they can just "get over" on their own.)
- Handout: Send them home with information that can be shared with parents. (Of course, parents have received information ahead of time too.)

Day 2 (1 hour):

- At the start of the session, hand out brief questionnaires that ask:
    o What is one thing you learned during the last session?
    o What is one thing you learned that surprised you?
    o What is one thing you learned that you already knew?
    o What questions or concerns do you still have?
        (We have found it is particularly helpful to have a trainer read through the cards while another trainer continues with the class to make sure all concerns are addressed before the students leave.)
- Review information from the previous session, and clear up any confusion or concerns. (There are often lingering questions that students are reluctant to ask out loud.)

- Have a discussion (with video clips, if available). (Reputable national organizations offer excellent videos. We *strongly suggest* you use one of these video clips, or another that has been vetted by a reputable suicide prevention organization. Well-meaning organizations that promote videos of true-life stories of suicidal teens, or of people who have died by suicide, can result in students who overidentify with the people in the video, which can escalate risk.)
  - o There are organizations that offer videos or video clips for classroom use, and they are listed below. (There are others. We simply recommend that you use a reputable suicide prevention organization when you select your videos for classroom use).

    Jed Foundation & MTVU ("Half of Us"), a free mental health literacy program to help teens feel less alone and encourage them to reach out (http://www.halfofus.com)

    American Foundation for Suicide Prevention (AFSP; "More Than Sad"), a video series with facilitator handbooks that has taught more than a million K–12 staff, students, and parents how to recognize, and intervene, when a young person might be suicidal (https://afsp.org/more-than-sad)

    Jed Storytellers (YouTube videos), a collection of mental health and suicide prevention campaigns for adolescents and young adults (https://www.youtube.com/user/TheJedFoundation)

- Role play—how to reach out to a friend. (We sometimes have a few students practice this at the front before all students pair up to practice this on their own.)

- Generate list: What adults could you talk to?
  - o If the school has adopted a particular slogan or logo for adults who are open to these difficult discussions, this is the time to tell students to look for the posted sign that says "You Can Talk to Me" (or whatever the school-specific slogan

might be) posted on the walls of teachers and staff who encourage these conversations. (We ask students to name specific people/roles in the school building of people they could approach. We are careful not to impose our assumptions, although we are often a bit concerned at how difficult it is for students to create this list in some schools!)

- Make sure all questions are answered before the students leave class. (Provide students with a way to have follow-up questions answered, after the training is over.)
- Provide all students with phone numbers for local suicide help and hotline. (Cards with the national number, 988, are often available from local resources, but cards with the local number can be made by running business card stock through a printer. We have found that it is particularly helpful to tell all students to take out their purses/wallets/backpacks and put these cards in them or, if they have their phones, to take a picture of this resource. That way, there is no stigmatizing effects that differentiate students who make a visible effort to keep the cards versus those who throw them away.)

In our work with schools, we have found that students respond well to this general format. Evaluations of the program are consistently positive at the end of training. Sample comments from participants (grades 8–12) at one of these trainings appear below.

- What is one main point or message that you have taken from these two presentations?
  - Suicide is never the answer.
  - We have to actually do something if a friend confronts us with suicide and not to keep it bottled up.
  - Suicide has so much effect on others.
  - You should talk to people close to you when they seem to be going through a tough time or have not acted normally.
  - Talk to others about your feelings.

- That suicide is a large problem but I have the power to help.
- That you always have someone to turn to; you can always get help.
- Suicide is a permanent solution to a temporary problem.
- That no matter what, you need to tell adults.
- Suicide is not worth it. You can always get help.
- Get help for yourself, and get help if you need it.
- It takes a strong person to help a friend thinking about suicide.
- Communication is probably the most important suicide prevention activity to do.
- Do you think, because of these presentations, you view suicide/depression or anyone dealing with suicide and/or depression differently? How?
  - Yes, I need to act quickly and take every word seriously if a person says they will commit suicide.
  - Yes, I feel after being presented with some of these statistics that I would like to change them for the better.
  - No, I have always been willing to help those dealing with these issues and myself have been diagnosed with manic depression.
  - Yes, because I know to be quick in getting help for someone considering suicide. I know not to keep it a secret.
  - I don't think those people are weird anymore. They are normal kids. This could happen to anyone.
  - Yes, I used to think they were crazy and they actually wanted to die, but now I know that they just want help. I should help them. Now I know how.
  - Yes, I see that suicide is preventable if you look for the warning signs.
  - Yes, I learned that depression is a disease that you can recover from.
  - Yes. I know it is very important to be open about this topic.

- Yes. Having examined the idea, it seems less likely that suicide is an answer.

Parent Education

Of course, it doesn't make any sense to tell young people that they need to tell an adult if they believe a friend is suicidal if the adults in their world don't know what to do with that information. We have seen far too many examples of adults who hear from their children that they are concerned about one of their friends or classmates, and the adults simply don't know what to do. *All* parents and guardians need information and education too. Whether that training occurs face to face at parent meetings or through information in newsletters or parent updates, it is important that parents know what to do if their child tells them about their own or another student's suicidal thoughts.

In some schools, we get access to parents though face-to-face meetings, although this is quite rare and never includes all parents. In other schools, we have access through newsletters and websites. We have found that it is essential to give information to parents periodically and in as many different formats as available. Face-to-face trainings can be similar in format and style to the gatekeeper training that we use for staff education and training, with additional emphasis on the importance of means restriction in the household (e.g., locking up guns and limiting access to pills or other potentially lethal methods). Information for newsletters and websites needs to be provided in engaging, short, and readable news briefs. Some schools offer a column on student mental health in every newsletter. Other schools offer information only periodically. We encourage schools to include information on mental health and suicide prevention in newsletters or other communications that go out during particularly stressful times for students, such as during exams, when college acceptance letters are being received, or before graduation. School websites should have an ongoing resource page for mental health. Regardless of the format, parents need to be given reliable and accurate information about suicide risk, mental health, and protective factors for their children.

Parents in particular need information about suicide myths, what they can do if they think there is a problem with their child, referral resources for assistance, and information on what kind of assistance is available. Just as with training for staff and students, parents need to be reminded that the most important thing they can do is *ask the question* and then *listen to the answer.*

Once parents have been given information, they will need to be alerted right before the suicide prevention education of their children occurs. We give parents a "heads up" that their child may come home with questions or concerns after the training, or may want to talk with them about a peer the student believes may be at risk. In general, the goal is to keep all lines of communication open.

Engage Peers With Peer Education

There is power in using students to help educate and inform students about suicide prevention. Teenagers are more likely to seek help if they believe their peers are supportive of mental health or if they have been encouraged by their friends to get help.

Several schools have made inroads in this effort by providing advanced training to some students, essentially making them "safe" peers who are one more resource to help at-risk students access the resources they need (Fulginati et al., 2016). Sometimes, these peer leaders receive advanced training, perhaps even a form of the suicide prevention gatekeeper training that is more typically offered to the staff and teachers. More often, peer leaders are engaged to help alter the social norms and acceptability of help seeking, essentially becoming the change agents of the school (Wyman et al., 2010). Orygen is a nonprofit organization from Australia that helps young people learn how to engage in safe digital communication about suicide (https://orygen.org.au).

Other schools have connected to larger peer education approaches. One example is Ohio's *Be Present Campaign*. This campaign gives young people knowledge and skills in suicide prevention. It is a student-led social media and marketing campaign (with much support and assistance from trained and involved adults). The goal is to teach students how to be leaders and advocates within their school buildings (for more information see https://bepresento hio.org).

Practical strategy (schools): We have found that helping student leaders find a way to take on additional roles within the school as peer advocates is helpful for several reasons. First, students often learn from, and model, their peers. Second, in any school building, just as with staff and teachers, there are a group of student leaders who want to be more involved in suicide prevention initiatives. Unless we help shape their behaviors through more advanced training, we have found that they will often become "de facto peer leaders," without that training (or with information that they learn on their own), with mixed results. It is far better that we bring them into our initiative.

General Strategies to Create a Culture of Care

In addition to training, most schools find that there are other strategies that are useful in developing a whole-school culture of care for suicide prevention. When suicide prevention is integrated into existing (or enhanced) school-wide approaches that promote student mental health rather than siloed as an "afterthought," the suicide prevention strategy is far more effective and meaningful (Jed Foundation, 2021). A comprehensive, public health approach to promote health, including mental health, well-being, and resilience, aims at supporting all students. Using this lens, all efforts to improve the well-being of the students in the school, to help students feel connected to the broader school environment, and to help reduce stigma for help seeking are clearly part of this larger culture of care.

Each school building will clearly have its own strategies and approaches that fit within the community, culture, and context. Programs, activities, and campaigns that promote connectiveness and belonging are important. Special attention should be paid to marginalized and high-risk groups, making extra efforts to bring them into the school community and to be intentional about the desire for the school to have a positive and inclusive school climate.

> *Practical strategy (schools): A trauma-informed school environment that promotes mental health and destigmatizes help seeking is an important strategy that helps promote a safe space where all students feel supported and included. One component of trauma-informed schools is teaching mental health literacy, framing treatment as one approach on a continuum of health-promoting strategies. This has been found to be more effective than simply teaching students about mental health diagnoses and treatment (McGorry et al., 2019).*

Although we cannot discuss every strategy to build this culture in this text, we offer a few suggestions below, which are based on our own work as well as our interactions with mental health professionals in the schools where we work. These have not been empirically validated but are offered only as a starting place for your own thinking. We encourage you to continue to reach out to other school mental health professionals, at conferences, over networking sites, or on your professional association websites, to share even more ideas. In additional, the National School Climate Center offers ideas and suggestions to get you thinking (http://www.school climate.org):

- "High-Five Fridays." At one school where we have trained, the school counselor stated that in her middle school, students, staff, and teachers make a point of giving "high fives"—and compliments—to each other every Friday. It is a way to make everyone in the building feel visible and acknowledged before the start of the weekend.
- "Mindfulness Mondays." Another school starts the week with this approach, helping students get into the right head-space for the start of the week. Rather than ending morning announcements in a rush, leaving students (and teachers) feeling frenzied and stressed, a moment of relaxation and deep breathing can help set the tone for the start of the day and the week.
- "Wall of Happiness." Students write happiness "graffiti" that changes every 2 weeks.
- "Positive People Group." A group of student leaders randomly leave Post-it® notes with positive messages around the school building.
- "Gratitude Board." Provide places in the hallways *and* the teachers' lounge where people can post notes expressing their gratitude for each other's actions.
- "30 Days of Kindness Challenge." Challenge all members of the school to perform 30 acts of kindness in 30 days.
- "Culture Club." Expose students to food, language, and experiences of people from different cultures. Have students (staff, teachers, and parents too!) from those cultures help lead the way and become the guides.
- "Student Ambassador Program." Recruit current students to act as guides and mentors for students who are new to the building.
- "Take a Break Station." Place these stations around the building and in almost every classroom. This allows students who recognize that they are not ready to learn because they feel stressed or overwhelmed to go to a specific place to calm

down and refocus. Ultimately, this helps build and reinforce essential self-monitoring skills that are useful for a lifetime.

The point is, there are many different ways that schools can help build a positive climate that helps students, staff, and teachers feel connected. Creating school-specific rituals and traditions that are fun and meaningful for students, staff, and teachers can be simple and cost-effective. For example, the first day of each month might have a special tradition that everyone comes to expect and enjoy.

Engage Peers With Student Organizations and Networks

We have found that when schools begin to pay attention to suicide prevention in meaningful ways, there are often groups of students who want to be more involved in suicide prevention and mental health promotion. It is important to engage these students. Finding substantial and valuable ways to help them be involved is crucial for creating the culture of care that is being developed in the building. We also know that students need mentoring, guidance, and support to engage in suicide prevention and mental health efforts in appropriate ways; we have our own experiences with both high school and college students trying to do good things to support suicide prevention that were clearly not well thought through.

Practical strategy (schools): Shape and guide your student groups. Rather than tell you how to do this, we will offer two cautionary tales. First, you may have heard of the "semicolon project." People receive semicolon tattoos to remind them that when the author comes to the end of a sentence, they can choose to stop, or they can choose to use a semicolon and continue. In this metaphor, you are the author, and the semicolon represents your decision to continue with your life, rather than to die by suicide. Each year, our University's

Campus Suicide Prevention Program purchases thousands of temporary semicolon tattoos to give out on Semicolon Day to share this powerful message. One year, a student group arranged to have an actual tattoo artist on campus, permanently tattooing our students for free—a kind gesture to be sure, but one that we could not support. I could not imagine the calls that I would receive from parents angry that we were sponsoring these impulsive (permanent) tattoos for their child.

The second story also happened at college. Several college students decided to raise money and awareness for suicide prevention after the death of actor Robin Williams, who died by suicide. It was a good and noble idea, but they decided to raise funds through a pub crawl. I learned of this when they tried to present our Campus Suicide Prevention Program with a check. I could only imagine the negative press our program would receive. The students had good intentions, but without mentoring and support, they did not understand why this was inappropriate. It was a difficult situation. The money was raised in good faith, and yet, we could not, in good faith, accept it. (The solution was to have them purchase something we needed and donate it to us, which kept us at arm's length from the funds.) Nevertheless, had we known about either of these scenarios ahead of time, we could have turned them both into learning experiences for the students and shaped their behavior. Instead, in both cases, we were left scrambling, and students were left feeling disgruntled and a bit unappreciated for their efforts.

There are many positive and proactive student activities and events that help empower students to engage in positive messaging and support around suicide prevention and mental health promotion. Student clubs help develop student leaders around these important topics. Community partners often provide important resources and assistance for these student activities too. There are so many ways that student groups can help change and enhance the culture of a school. Students who participate in these types of clubs and activities have significant reductions in their mental health stigma and more willingness to seek help for themselves and others (Pescosolido, 2019). We offer just a few suggestions below, but there are many others.

- Out of the Darkness Walk for Suicide Prevention. The American Foundation for Suicide Prevention hosts walks each year in many communities throughout the United States. Student clubs often sponsor teams in these walks, promoting mental health and suicide prevention (https://afsp.org).
- Active Minds. This national organization focuses on student advocacy for mental health. Although it was traditionally for college students, there are now chapters in over 100 high schools. Active Minds is very involved in legislative advocacy and student leadership development. Their most recognized campaign is the Send Silence Packing program, which is a traveling exhibit of backpacks that represent young lives lost to suicide each year (http://www.activeminds.org).
- Bring Change to Mind (BC2M). This mental health club for high school students helps promote healthy ways to manage stress. One popular activity, Little Worries, helps students recognize that they are not alone in their struggles (http://bring change2mind.org).
- National Alliance on Mental Illness. Traditionally, this organization was designed for individuals who have, or who have friends or family with, mental health conditions. The goal of the club is to create a safe and inclusive school environment (https://www.nami.org).

Practical strategy (schools): For years, the Suicide Prevention Program at the Ohio State University has been running an annual RU OK? Day. This day is led by a student group (with support and mentoring from our staff) and is a large-scale effort to teach students, staff, and faculty on our university campus to ask this important question. As members of our campus community enter a very large ballroom space, they are given a card with the four letters and question mark. As they move to each area of the room, they encounter students who provide education and information (R = resources in the community, U = university resources, O = organizations that support students, K = cultural and specialized supports, and? = how to ask the question). Once they have learned this important information, they have their card punched. A completed card is worth a free t-shirt that says RU OK? This model has been adopted by several high schools that we have worked with. Students are eager to use this approach to teach their classmates, local businesses are often happy to donate t-shirts associated with this positive messaging, and best of all, at the end, students walk around the building for weeks and months to come with shirts sporting a message of caring and inclusivity. The Ohio States University Suicide Prevention Program website has images and information about this student-led initiative (http://www.suicidepre vention.osu.edu).

Conclusion

Once schools have developed a comprehensive suicide prevention plan, the next step is implementation. For most schools, school mental health professionals will require some advanced preparation and training in suicide assessment and intervention first. Once there are members of the school who are prepared to assist with suicidal students, the next step involves training the staff and teachers. All adults who interact with students should be confident, competent, and willing to interact with suicidal students and to refer them to the appropriate staff in the school building. To do this, everyone will require training that enhances their knowledge, beliefs, attitudes, skills, and self-efficacy. Schools should also prepare parents so they know how to speak with their children who either express suicidal ideation themselves or voice concerns about their friends.

Students will require developmentally appropriate education. For younger grades, this means social and emotional learning that gives them skills that prepare them for a lifetime of coping. For students in older grades, schools may decide to engage in suicide prevention education. Students in older grades may also in engage in peer education and suicide prevention activities and outreach, with appropriate staff mentoring and support.

References

Albright, G., Adam, C., Serri, D., Bleeker, S., & Goldman, R. (2016). Harnessing the power of conversations with virtual humans to change health behaviors. *mHealth, 6*(2), 1–13. doi:10.21037/mhealth.2016.11.02

Aseltine, R. H., Jr., James, A., Schilling, E. A., & Glanovsky, T. (2007). Evaluating the SOS suicide prevention program: A replication and extension. *BMC Public Health, 7*, 161. doi:10.1186/1471-2458-7-16-1

Doan, J., Roggenbaum, S., Lazear, K. J., & LeBlanc, A. (2012). *Youth suicide prevention school-based guide—Issue brief 3b: Risk factors: How can a school identify a student at risk for suicide.* University of South Florida, College of Behavioral and Community Sciences, Louis de la Parte Florida Mental Health Institute, Department of Child & Family Studies (FMHI Series Publication #218-3b-Rev 2012).

Dray, J., Bowman, J., Campbell, E., Freund, M., Wolfenden, L., Hodder, R. K., McElwaine, K., Tremain, D., Bartlem, K., Bailey, J., Small, T., Palazzi, K., Oldmeadow, C., & Wiggers, J. (2017). Systematic review of universal resilience-focused interventions targeting child and adolescent mental health in the school setting. *Journal of the American Academy of Child and Adolescent Psychiatry, 56*(10), 813–824.

Fulginati, A., Rice, E., Hsu, H. T., Rhoades, H., & Winetrobe, H. (2016). Risky integration: A social network analysis of network position, exposure, and suicidal ideation among homeless youth. *Journal of Crisis Intervention and Suicide Prevention, 37*(3), 184–193.

Hazelden. (2018). *Lifelines Prevention Curriculum.* Author.

Isaac, M., Elias, B., Katz, L. Y., Belik, S. L., Deane, F. P., Enns, M. W., Sareen, J., & Swampy Cree Suicide Prevention Team. (2009). Gatekeeper training as a preventative intervention for suicide: A systematic review. *Canadian Journal of Psychiatry, 54,* 260–268.

Jed Foundation. (2021). *A comprehensive approach to mental health promotion and suicide prevention for high schools.* http://jedfoundation.org

Juhnke, G. A., Granello, D. H., & Granello, P. F. (2011). *Suicide, self-injury, and violence in the schools: Assessment, prevention, and intervention strategies.* Wiley.

McGorry, P., Trethowan, J., & Rickwood, D. (2019). Creating headspace for integrated youth mental health care. *World Psychiatry, 18*(2), 140–141.

National Action Alliance for Suicide Prevention: Research Prioritization Task Force. (2014). *A prioritized research agenda for suicide prevention: An action plan to save lives.* National Institute of Mental Health.

Pescosolido, B. A., Perry, B. L., & Krendl, A. C. (2019). Empowering the next generation to end stigma by starting the conversation: Bring change to mind and the college toolbox project. *Journal of the American Academy of Child & Adolescent Psychiatry, 59*(4), 519–530. doi:10.1016/j.jaac.2019.06.016

SAVE.org. (2021). *Linking education and awareness of depression and suicide (LEADS).* http://save.org.

Schmidt, R. C. (2016). Mental health practitioners' perceived levels of preparedness, levels of confidence and methods used in the assessment of youth suicide risk. *Professional Counselor, 6*(1), 76–88.

Sheftall, A. H., Asti, L., Horowitz, L. M., Felts, A., Fontanella, C. A., Campo, J. V., & Bridge, J. A. (2016). Suicide in elementary school-aged children and early adolescents. *Pediatrics, 138*(4), 1–10. doi:10.1542/peds.2016-0436

Sheftall, A. H., Bergdoll, E. E., James, M., Bauer, C., Spector, E., Vakil, R., Armstrong, E., Allen, J., & Bridge, J. A. (2020). Emotion regulation in elementary school-aged children with a maternal history of suicidal behavior: A pilot study. *Child Psychiatry and Human Development, 51*(5), 792–800. doi:10.1007/s10578-020-01010-8

Singer, J. B., & Slovak, K. (2011). School social workers' experiences with youth suicidal behavior: An exploratory study. *Children & Schools, 33,* 215–228.

Substance Abuse Mental Health Services Administration. (2012). *Preventing suicide: A toolkit for high schools.* U.S. Department of Health and Human Services.

Wilcox, H. C., Kellam, S. G., Brown, C. H., Poduska, J., Ialongo, N. S., Wang, W., & Anthony, J. C. (2008). The impact of two universal randomized first and second grade classroom interventions on young adult suicide ideation and attempt. *Drug and Alcohol Dependence, 95*(Suppl. 1), S60–S73. doi:10.1016/j.drugalcdep.2008.01.005

Wyman, P. A., Brown, C. H., LoMurray, M., Schmeelk-Cone, K., Petrova, M., Yu, Q., Walsh, E., Tu, X., & Wang, W. (2010). An outcome evaluation of the

Sources of Strength suicide prevention program delivered by adolescent peer leaders in high schools. *American Journal of Public Health, 100*(9), 1653–1661. doi:10.2105/AJPH.2009.l90025

Yonemoto, N., Kawashima, Y., Endo, K., & Yamada, M. (2019). Gatekeeper training for suicidal behaviors: A systematic review. *Journal of Affective Disorders, 246,* 506–514.

8

Assessing Suicide Risk in Schools

On any day, in any middle or high school across the United States, nearly 1 in 5 students is walking around the building having seriously thought about killing themselves within this last year. In the postpandemic world, about 1 in 10 has seriously thought about suicide in just this last month (Czeisler et al., 2020). As you walk through the halls of your school building today, stop for a moment. Every 12th child that you encounter carries with them the knowledge that they have had a suicide attempt this past year. And today, over 5,000 kids will try to take their own lives.

The ability to recognize, intervene, and refer these students to appropriate care is one of the most complex and challenging skills that most school-based mental health professionals must perform. It is also undoubtedly one of the most important. There are no easy answers, and there are no shortcuts. In this chapter we will provide you with the most up-to-date information and resources to help you with this important task. We also hope you recognize that this is a skill that requires more than book training. We encourage you to seek additional education, support, and supervision, particularly if you have not received adequate training in these skills before. Even if you have received training and are skilled in this task, suicide risk assessment is something that always requires consultation and collaboration.

In the previous two chapters (Chapters 6 and 7), we discussed tier one, or **universal intervention**, a school-wide approach to suicide prevention. In this chapter and the next, we turn our attention to the next two levels of support. **Selective intervention** (also called

Suicide and Self-Injury in Schools. Darcy Haag Granello, Paul F. Granello, Gerald A. Juhnke,
Oxford University Press. © Oxford University Press 2023. DOI: 10.1093/oso/9780190059842.003.0008

tier two) is for groups of students who are identified as needing extra support, often through an informal assessment. **Indicated intervention** (tier three) is for students who are suicidal and require individual assistance.

Suicidal students require special attention in schools. We recognize that although most school mental health personnel want desperately to help suicidal students, these students can be challenging to manage within the constraints of the school setting. They represent a significant drain on school resources and staff time. Even more importantly, we know that these students can be emotionally difficult for those who work with them. There are often very real limits to what we can do and how we can help. Nevertheless, whether or not any of us want the responsibility of managing this difficult population to fall to our already overburdened and underfunded schools, we don't have a choice. These students are in the building, and they need our help.

Practical strategy (self): We know that working with suicidal students is stressful. In our work, we have found that there are some very common emotional reactions, including the following:

- *Fear*
- *Anxiety*
- *Anger*
- *Hopelessness*
- *Helplessness*

We encourage you to stop and think for a moment about your own reactions to working with these students. The reactions that are listed might resonate with you—and you might have others. It is important to take time to recognize your emotional response. Your own reactions may influence what you do, the decisions you make, and how you engage in suicide risk assessments. For example, based on the emotional reactions you have, you might be more likely to be

- *overprotective (fear every student is at risk, sound the alarm for every student that anyone is even slightly concerned about before the concern is fully explored, not allow the student to engage in any developmentally appropriate strategies for self-care, impose overly restrictive environments and external controls),*
- *disengaged (so anxious or stressed out about the situation that you do not fully engage with the students or parents and are eager to refer the student to the next level of care because you feel overwhelmed), or*
- *resigned (so overwhelmed by the magnitude of the problem that you feel unable to do anything about it, convinced that no matter what we do, students will make their own choices about suicide, parents will either be engaged or not, and there is little point in being proactive).*

Of course, there are positive reactions to working with these students too. Most school mental health professionals also feel a positive sense of purpose and meaning when they can help save the lives of the students in their care. We recognize, support, and value the commitment you are making to your students, and we don't want to focus only on the negative. We know from years of experience working with school personnel, however, that it is these common negative emotional reactions that are more difficult to process out loud. School mental health professionals tell us (in private) that they feel embarrassed or ashamed that they have these negative reactions. We understand. This is complicated work. Taking a moment to acknowledge within yourself that you can have both positive and negative reactions to working with suicidal students is important. Giving yourself permission to stay with those negative emotions for a moment might actually improve your skills. We hope it helps to know that others share these complex emotions.

Even those who recognize the importance of the task of assessing and managing suicidal students in schools can feel a bit overwhelmed by the magnitude of the need and the seriousness of the responsibility. Suicidal students need intensive and extensive care. Comprehensive suicide risk assessments require advanced clinical skills and experience, and that is clearly beyond what can typically be offered within the school environment. So too the ongoing management of highly suicidal students is challenging. Clearly, there are inherent limitations to the amount and type of mental health services that schools can provide to suicidal students. Most schools do not have a sufficient number of trained mental health professionals in the building to offer the type of care that these students need. Few schools meet the recommended ratios for school counselors or school psychologists, and many schools do not have a school nurse or social worker in the building at all.

Nevertheless, in spite of the challenges, schools offer unparalleled access to youth to recognize when students might be at risk for suicide and to begin the process of risk assessment. Schools also offer students excellent access to caring adults and resources to help prevent suicide. In addition, as we discussed in the last two chapters, schools can reduce the stigma associated with mental illness and help seeking and can promote a healthy approach to wellness and support.

Selective Interventions: Identifying Students Who Need Extra Support

Selective interventions provide services for groups of students who are at elevated risk. In general, these services either address existing risk factors or build protective factors in groups of students with behavioral and/or mental health problems who are not at immediate risk for suicide. Of course, these groups of students will, by definition, have been exposed to any universal prevention programming that has already occurred in the school. However, the information contained in that universal approach may not have been of sufficient dosage or focus for these specific vulnerable populations. Thus, selective interventions provide additional information, training, and support to these identified groups.

Many selective intervention strategies are linked to more advanced training designed to increase students' social and emotional competence, with the recognition that these students are typically operating from a deficit in this area. In this way, although selective intervention programs are intended to help *prevent* suicide, they can really be thought of as early *intervention* strategies. That is, groups of students are given additional assistance at more intense levels than is typically part of a school's suicide prevention program. The goal is to move them from a place of elevated risk back to within the behaviors and boundaries of the "typical" or "average" student population.

Selective interventions require an understanding of what groups might be at elevated risk and a mechanism to determine which students fall into these high-risk groups. Selective prevention strategies focus specifically on seeking out these youth and proactively offering them additional services and care. In general, these strategies are expected to impact the approximately 20% of youth who are at high risk for developing suicidal behaviors.

Practical strategy (schools): There are many ways to help students learn how to improve their emotional self-regulation. One strategy that is gaining momentum is the use of S.M.A.R.T (Stress Management and Resiliency Training) Labs. These labs offer biofeedback using HeartMath® technology, helping students to manage emotional dysregulation. In pilot studies, S.M.A.R.T. Labs at the middle and high school level, as well as at universities, demonstrated significant improvements across a variety of measures. For example, 745 middle school students who participated in a S.M.A.R.T. Lab for an average of 23 minutes per student saw significant improvement (18%, higher, on average) in Heart Rate Variability (HRV). Higher HRV correlates to better psychological health as well as a greater ability to adapt to change and stress. Middle school students (n=78) who engaged in group activities using the S.M.A.R.T. Lab as a selective intervention saw a 19% improvement in G.P.A. and an average decrease of 25 school absences over the course of a year. Middle school students who were identified as at significantly elevated risk for suicide (indicated intervention) who participated in a S.M.A.R.T. Lab (n=22) had, on average, 4 fewer behavioral incidents, moving from an average of 8 per year to 4 (https://smartlabconsultants.com). In other words, concentrated efforts to help students learn to self-regulate their emotions, in this case with the assistance of biofeedback, can significantly improve outcomes for students at all levels of risk.

Assessing Students for Selective Interventions

There is no specific assessment instrument that is used to identify students who might benefit from selective interventions. Some of the students who might benefit may already be known to school personnel. This is particularly likely if school staff, teachers, and parents are taught to identify troubled students, as discussed in the previous chapter. Students who have learned to tell a trusted adult if they are concerned about a friend or peer might also alert school personnel of students who might benefit from selective interventions. Additionally, teachers can be asked to identify and refer students who are displaying problematic behaviors in the classroom. Such behaviors might include impulsivity, hopelessness, or withdrawal. Finally, students who have been brought to the attention of mental health professionals and received a suicide risk assessment and found not to be at imminent risk for suicide might benefit from selective interventions.

Many of the positive and prosocial interventions that are intended to promote mental health that school counselors, school psychologists, school social workers, and school nurses provide are all forms of selective intervention. Whenever students begin to display problematic behaviors or have risk factors due to biological predispositions or psychological vulnerabilities, they could benefit from selective interventions. Students who are at risk because of their histories, identities, living situations, environmental context, or treatment at the hands of their peers also could benefit. For example, when elementary-aged children with no friends are singled out to join a psychoeducational group to teach them social skills, this can provide the kind of protective factors that can ultimately help buffer against suicide risk. When middle school special education students who exhibit problems with aggression and anger are put on a behavioral management plan to limit their angry outbursts and to get their needs met in more appropriate ways, this can be a form of selective intervention. When high school males who are isolated and withdrawn are given wallet cards with the local suicide hotline number, this also is a form of selective intervention. In other words, whenever a student is identified as being part of a group at high risk for mental health problems and an effort is made to intervene, this is selective intervention.

Using this broad definition for selective intervention means that many of the programs and activities in schools meet the criteria for inclusion under this umbrella. However, the inclusion of so many programs and interventions makes assessment of the effectiveness of these programs, specifically as they relate to suicide risk, nearly impossible to determine. Nevertheless, other measures of outcomes, including reduced behavioral problems, improved functioning, higher levels of connectedness to the school, and lowered stigma for help seeking, all are correlated with reduced risk for suicide.

Indicated Interventions: Identifying Suicidal Students

Students require an immediate indicated intervention once they are identified as potentially suicidal. As soon as these students come to the attention of school staff, the appropriate school mental health professional must conduct an initial suicide risk assessment within the same school day and facilitate a referral as necessary.

In this section, we will guide you through the process of identifying these students and conducting a school-based risk assessment. We will also assist with helping you develop protocols for this process. In the next chapter, we will discuss the process of intervening with these students, including facilitating referrals, interacting with parents, and managing the student's mental health.

Developing a Risk Assessment Protocol

Before any potentially suicidal student comes to the attention of school mental health professionals, there must be clear policies and guidelines in place of how a suicide risk assessment will be handled. We *strongly encourage* all schools to have clear and explicit steps to follow that are developed *before* a crisis. We offer some overall guidance, based on our work and in compliance with a model policy developed by the American Foundation for Suicide Prevention (AFSP, 2019), in coordination with the American School Counselor Association (ASCA), the National Association of School Psychologists (NASP), and the Trevor Project. ASCA has an additional policy to help school counselors navigate the challenge of suicide risk assessment (2020).

- Create a crisis response team of trained mental health professionals who will immediately intervene with a potentially suicidal student.
  - o Within that team, identify a trained school-based mental health professional who is the designated assessor and will lead the suicide assessment. Whenever possible, having a second trained mental health professional included in the assessment is ideal. Have clear protocols in place for who

will conduct the assessment if the primary identified assessor is unavailable.

o In schools where there is no mental health professional in place, identify a staff person who will address the situation according to policy until a trained mental health professional is brought in.

- Continuously supervise any potentially suicidal student to ensure safety until the assessment process is complete.

o This means that a staff person or teacher should escort the student to the appropriate staff person. Never "send" the student on their own.

o Potentially suicidal students should never be allowed to be alone, not even to use the restroom.

o Under no circumstances should the student be allowed to leave the school without appropriate supervision (e.g., parent, police, emergency medical technician).

- If the student currently has the means to carry out the suicide (e.g., gun, knife), seek voluntary relinquishment, but *do not force the student to do so and do not place yourself in danger.*

- Keep the student informed of all of the decisions that are being made and people who are being notified.

- Identify which administrators must be notified (e.g., principal, Suicide Prevention Coordinator, crisis response coordinator) and notify immediately.

- In the case of an in-school attempt, the health and safety of the student are paramount.

o Render first aid, following school protocols, until professional medical treatment and/or transportation is available.

o Supervise/stay with the student to ensure safety.

o Move all other students out of the immediate area as soon as possible.

- Conduct a suicide risk assessment.

o Consult with school staff and teachers, as appropriate, for corroborating information.

- o Determine level of risk to develop an action plan. However, use caution not to categorize this risk as "low, medium, or high"—as this can oversimplify the situation.
- Contact the parent or guardian, in accordance with state law and district policy.
  - o If the parent or guardian is deemed to escalate risk or in cases of suspected abuse, contact Child Protective Services.
  - o Regardless of risk level, work with caregivers to remove lethal means, such as guns, poisons, medications, and sharp objects, or to limit their accessibility.
  - o Refer to community services, as appropriate.
  - o Request that guardians sign a release of information to discuss the student's health with outside care, if appropriate.
- Develop a strategy for student safety/management within the school building.
  - o Intervention strategies and safety management must occur whether the student remains in school or returns after emergency care.
- Document all interactions and all decisions.
  - o Schools are legally responsible for documenting every step in the assessment and intervention process.
- Continue to monitor the school climate and other students for possible contagion effects.

Practical strategy (schools): Whenever possible, it is ideal to have two trained school-based mental health professionals conduct the school-based suicide risk assessment. We recognize that this is not always possible. However, we know that it can be extremely useful to have one person attend to the physical (safety) and emotional needs of the student, while the other is more focused on the actual risk assessment, including the logistics of notifying guardians, administrators, and (when necessary) emergency personnel. In addition, we know from experience that during times of heightened crisis, having another trained professional means

*another person who might hear or see things that another might
overlook.*

Student Referrals

Students will come to the attention of school mental health
professionals as needing a school-based suicide risk assessment
through a variety of sources. Anyone in the school system might
express concern about the student, including a peer, a staff person,
a teacher, or an administrator. In addition, students might come
forward themselves for help.

Staff and Teacher Referrals. In the previous chapter, we
discussed how to train staff and teachers to recognize students
who might be at risk for suicide and mental health distress.
Staff and teachers who have been trained as suicide prevention
gatekeepers and who know what to do and how to intervene are
more likely to recognize students in distress and reach out and
get them appropriate care. Whether staff or teachers have received this training, however, school mental health professionals
can encourage everyone in the building to let them know if they
are particularly concerned about the mental health of one of the
students.

*Practical strategy (schools): Most school counselors or other school
mental health professionals use referral forms so staff or teachers can
refer students who might be experiencing behavioral or emotional
problems. Differentiating between students who are at risk for suicide and need to be walked to the counselor's office for a risk assessment and students who are escalating in problematic behaviors and
would benefit from a conversation with a counselor is important.
Teach staff and teachers to ask important questions, such as "Is this
a safety issue?" or "Has the student demonstrated any clear signs of
suicide, such as talking/writing about suicide, death, hopelessness, or*

*self-harm?" or "Has the student's behavior changed significantly over
the last few days?"*

Student and Self-Referrals. Students should be encouraged not
to keep secrets if they know a friend is at risk for suicide. Not only
might their friend die without professional help, but also there is
ample evidence that the student who kept the secret is at higher risk
for suicide if they knew this secret and didn't seek out help. Because
this can be a difficult conversation, anything that school mental
health professionals can do to encourage students to share information about potentially suicidal students with trusted adults is
helpful. A common approach, for example, is anonymous peer referral. We have heard from several students that they have used this
"reporting" system to seek help for themselves, stating that it was
easier to go to the counselor's office at the behest of an anonymous
report than it was to admit that they needed help.

Electronic Referrals. Many schools are now grappling with the
challenges of how to monitor students' online behaviors. Students
who discuss suicide and death in their social media platforms
may have this behavior reported by their peers. More and more
schools, however, are monitoring their students' online behavior.
Schools that embrace social media and/or Internet monitoring
argue that they are protecting the safety of their students. Others
worry that this type of surveillance has potential legal and ethical
implications (Cvek, 2017). In spite of the challenges, schools that
use this type of software (typically for both suicide and homicide
threats) often provide specific examples of lives saved, even as they
recognize the expense of these programs, both monetarily and in
staff time (Byars et al., 2020). Electronic monitoring also results
in many "false positives." For example, students studying *Romeo
and Juliet* may find that their keyword searches cause red flags in
the software. Nevertheless, schools that use this type of software
know that responding to a student in real time, 24/7, can make a
difference.

Practical strategy (schools): It is important to determine who will monitor the alerts of student electronic media during off-school times, if schools choose to participate in this type of electronic surveillance. Many of these alerts come in late at night—sometimes in the middle of the night—and they must be addressed immediately in order to be effective. Clearly, this places an enormous burden on these staff members, who must be appropriately trained to recognize level of risk and to know what to do. They must also receive appropriate support, flex time, and compensation.

Suicide Risk Assessment Interviews

There is *no standardized method or assessment tool* that will determine which students will die by suicide. There are some checklists and assessments that will help, and we'll get to those in a moment. However, the first and most important step is always to simply talk with the student. Without solid rapport and a clear understanding of what the student is feeling, the assessment instruments are likely to be ineffective. Assessment interviews, however, are not just free-form conversations. They are semistructured interviews that take students to specific areas of questioning in intentional ways designed to elicit information that will help determine risk. Coupled with checklists or other types of risk assessments, they can help guide the determination of next steps in the action plan.

Asking the Most Important Question. The first and most important component of a risk assessment is to *ask the suicide question directly.* Although it may be uncomfortable, it is important. Use the word "suicide" or "kill yourself." Stay away from questions like "Are you thinking of hurting yourself?" Although that is a fine question to assess self-harm, it is *not* the same as assessing for suicide. The reason is, there are students who believe that they have found a way to die that will not hurt, and they will answer "no" to this question, even though they fully intend to die. The question is simple: "Are you thinking of killing yourself?" or "Have you thought about suicide?" As follow-up questions, you might also try the following:

- "Have you ever wished you were dead?" (This assesses a more passive suicide intent.)
- "Have you ever thought your friends or family would be better off if you were dead?"
- "Have you thought about killing yourself in the past?"
- "Have you tried to kill yourself before?"

Sometimes people couch these questions in phrases such as "When people are really [upset, angry, hurting], they sometimes think about killing themselves. Is that something that you have thought about?" We think this is a fine question for students who have the cognitive capacity to understand the intent of this question. For *very young* or *extremely cognitively rigid* children, we have learned from our work that this may be a dangerous way to phrase this question. Young children often rely on adults to problem-solve for them, and a poorly worded question may imply that the adult is offering a "solution." We have found that by the time children have some reasoning capacity, this typically is no longer a problem and actually helps to normalize the thoughts (while taking care not to normalize the behaviors).

Within these general guidelines, the actual wording of the question is not terribly important. We encourage you to use language that makes sense for you and for the student you are assessing. We have found that when people get too worried about the exact wording of these questions, they can sound artificial or robotic, and that doesn't help rapport. Having the questions emerge more organically from you makes sense. Perhaps the only questions that we absolutely *do not* recommend are ones like these: "You're not thinking of killing yourself, are you?" or "You were just kidding about suicide, right?" Clearly, those types of questions do not open up lines of communication.

Using the word "suicide" is important. Students who are suicidal need to feel heard, understood, and validated. The word can feel frightening and overwhelming to them, and it is unfair to make them say it first. Having the adult use the word, and giving the student permission to say the word out loud, makes it feel less powerful. If the student is not feeling suicidal, then they will not say "yes." (There is *no truth* to the myth that talking about suicide will put the idea in someone's head.) But if they *are* thinking about suicide, the message that is communicated by using this word is that it is okay to talk about it, and suicide assessments work best when students believe they can communicate openly. In the words of one of the students we assessed:

> It was just such a relief to be able to say the word suicide out loud. I felt like everybody was avoiding the word when they talked to me, and it made me feel like I had to avoid it too. And that made me feel even more like there was something wrong with me. When you said suicide, it was like this big weight just came off my shoulders.

In our work with school personnel, we are surprised to learn that many never ask about suicide, even if they think a student might be at risk. Not long ago, we did a training of school staff on suicide risk assessment. About 90 minutes into the training, we called up several staff members for a role play. About 5 minutes in, when the person portraying a school staff member still had not used the word suicide, we stopped the role play and asked, "When are you going to ask about suicide?" The school staff person responded, "Oh, I would *never* ask about suicide in *real life*!" After all the training, the person still hadn't made the connection about the importance of asking the suicide question. Unfortunately, that reaction is all too common. The most important thing to do to assess suicide risk is to *ask the suicide question.*

Practical strategy (schools): This isn't just about asking the suicide question as a "yes/no" (although that is important). For some students, that short one-word answer (or head nod) is easiest. For others, the response is more complicated. A yes/no is too concrete—and <u>in addition to</u> the yes/no question, it is important to ask the question in a way that allows for more nuanced thinking ("Can you talk with me about any thoughts you are having about living versus dying?"). For other students, it is easier to write down their thoughts than it is to say them out loud. The point is, although we need to ask the suicide question of every student we assess, we also have to allow students other means to express their suicidal thoughts, if that is easier for them.

Of course, when students are asked the suicide question, they may respond with a "no"—even if they are suicidal. They may deny their suicidal thoughts and behaviors for many different reasons. Perhaps they don't want help, they don't trust the person they are speaking with, or they are fearful of what will happen next if they admit to these feelings. Therefore, it's important not to accept the first "no"—and to move forward with next steps in care regardless of the student's answer if there is reason to believe the student is at risk.

Practical strategy (schools): We discussed the importance of being "gently persistent" in Chapter 7, when we encouraged suicide prevention gatekeepers not to accept the first "no" when they asked students if they were suicidal. It is worth noting that being "gently persistent" is also important in suicide risk assessment. Remember that most people have been socially conditioned not to talk about suicide and to respond to questions about their well-being with responses like "I'm fine" or "I'm okay." We encourage you to stay with the student, to demonstrate your care and interest, and to give them time to answer your questions, even if this means asking it multiple times and in multiple ways.

Why Do This Assessment? Before we go any further, you might be thinking, "If the student says they are suicidal, that means I am going to call a parent, and they are going to be sent to an outside referral for a comprehensive risk assessment, so why am I asking any more questions?" Of course, in one way, you are right. School-based mental health professionals typically do *not* make the final determinations about level of suicide risk. Once there is an indication of risk, the protocol the school has in place for notifying parents and arranging for a referral for a risk assessment and other assistance for the student will begin. *However*, once the student has begun the conversation and revealed their suicidal thinking, eliciting more information, if possible, is important. Simply calling a parent the second a student mentions the word "suicide" doesn't help the student feel heard or supported. Yes, the parents need to be called within a few minutes, but clearly there will be a few follow-up questions and some moments to build empathy and support. Using those moments in a way that is productive is important. School mental health professionals provide crucial components of the risk assessment, and gaining information to pass along to parents and other mental health professionals (with releases signed, of course) is essential.

There are three Cs to risk assessment:

- **Collaboration:** School mental health professionals should work closely with parents and with clinicians in the community, helping to provide the best possible care for the student.
- **Corroboration:** If students share details and information about suicidal plans and intent, that information is important to pass along to parents and clinicians who are making final determinations of risk. It is not uncommon for students to tell pieces of the story to different people—and sharing those pieces can help create the larger context.

- **Consultation:** As we have repeatedly said, all of us are better at conducting risk assessments *at any level* when we work together and receive feedback, supervision, mentoring, and consultation on our work.

To this standard list of the three Cs that we use in our trainings, we could add a few more, including:

Counseling: Those who are conducting risk assessments should use their counseling skills to convey warmth, empathy, and unconditional positive regard (Rogers, 1957).

Confidentiality—although standard confidentiality protocols *do not exist* during times of self-harm, this does not mean that *everyone* in the school needs to know what is going on or be given confidential information about the student. Be judicious about who included in these discussions.

Complexity—suicide risk assessment is extraordinarily complex and challenging. Those who complete these assessments often follow some core principles to help guide the process. These are discussed in the following paragraphs.

Core Areas to Assess

In addition to asking the suicide question, there are three key components to assess that will help determine suicide risk: ideation, intent, and plan. Once these have been assessed, there is an opportunity to gather more details about risk factors, warning signs, and protective factors.

We ask students to tell us about their suicidal thoughts. Are they frequent? Are they becoming more frequent? When did they first notice these thoughts? What led up to the thoughts (e.g., interpersonal or intrapsychic antecedents)? How close have they come to acting on the thoughts in the past? How likely are they to act on them in the future? In general, the point here is to get students talking about their suicidal thoughts so we get a sense of the narrative surrounding these thoughts.

Suicide Ideation.   As students answer the suicide question, their level of ideation may well become apparent. Nevertheless, it is important to ask them, specifically, about their thoughts of suicide.

For most students, ideation occurs over time, and questions about thoughts of suicide typically ask about the *history* of the ideation. We might ask, for example, about ideation during the past 2 weeks, over the past month, over the past year, and at the present moment. We also want to know when the student first noticed these thoughts. Can they identify anything that led up to the thoughts (interpersonal or intrapsychic antecedents)?

Once the student acknowledges these thoughts, then we help them clarify the *frequency* of the thoughts: Every day? Every hour? Every minute? Has the frequency changed? Frequency of ideation helps understand risk.

Next, we want to understand the *intensity* of the thoughts: Can they continue to function? Are they unable to do anything else when the thoughts come? Can they change their thinking when the suicidal thoughts occur, or are they fixated on these thoughts? Intensity also helps us understand risk.

Finally, we ask about the *duration* of the thoughts: Are these just fleeting moments? Hours? All day? Duration also affects risk.

Taken together, the *history, frequency, intensity,* and *duration* of the suicide ideation all factor into understanding suicide risk. If the thoughts have changed significantly over the past few weeks or days, if they occur with changing and increasing frequency, if they are unable to think of anything else or stop themselves from obsessing about these thoughts, and if the thoughts are more than just fleeting, then clearly the risk of suicide increases.

Practical strategy (schools): Any time a student says they have "command hallucinations" of suicide (or violence of any sort), this automatically places them into a "suicide emergency" category.

Command hallucinations, although relatively rare among young people, are exceedingly dangerous and must be addressed immediately by experts in clinical settings.

Suicide Intent. Most people who are suicidal do not want to die. They want the unbearable psychological pain they are feeling to go away. Nevertheless, when students are hopeless and cannot imagine another way to end their pain, their likelihood of dying by suicide increases. Asking students about their intent on a scale of 1–5 (1 is "I don't want to die," 3 is "part of me wants to die," and 5 is "I want to die") is helpful. Younger students (or those with limited cognitive capacity) may benefit from a 1–3 scale, where there can be no confusion about what these numbers might mean (Erbacher et al., 2015).

Practical strategy (schools): We have found that McGlothlin's SIMPLE STEPS (2008) approach is particularly helpful for assessing intent. In this model, one of the questions is to ask students not only their current level of intent on a scale of 1–10 but also, importantly, "What would it take for you to get to a 10?" This helps us understand the student's level of volatility, or their capacity to cope. In other words, a student who currently assesses their intent as a 4 and has difficulty naming anything that would get them to a 10 clearly has a lower level of risk than a student who rates themselves a 4 but says a hostile text from a friend would get them to a 10. We use McGlothlin's scaling questions, with the caveat that with young people, we have found a 1–5 scale is often more appropriate than a 1–10 scale.

Suicide Plan. Understanding the student's suicide plan, if they have one, can help better assess risk. For example, we have had students say to us, when asked about a suicide plan, "I don't know. I would probably take some pills or something, or maybe jump into traffic." We also have had students say something like "I get home at 3:30; my parents don't get home until 6. I will call my mom to tell her I got home safe from school; otherwise she will check up on me. I will get my dad's gun. He keeps it locked up, but I know where the key is. I know how to load the bullets too. I will go into my bedroom, lock the door behind me, and shoot myself in the mouth." Clearly, the second scenario represents a student at higher imminent risk. In general, when assessing a suicide plan, we consider (a) details of the plan (the more details, the higher the risk); (b) intent (in general, students who fully intend to die are at higher risk than those who are more ambivalent); (c) means (more lethal means relates to higher risk); (d) access to means (easier access equals higher risk); and (e) proximity of help (the less likely that someone will intervene, the higher the risk). Remember, many suicidal students will withhold some information, and it is best to assume that they have done more than they are admitting. For example, if the student says they "might get some pills," it is quite likely they already have acquired some. In general, it is always better to err on the side of caution.

When students develop suicide plans, it is clear that it is the student's *intent* behind those plans that is important, not the actual lethality. Students who survive attempts only because they chose a nonlethal dosage or a nonfatal method will certainly learn and have a future attempt or completion. We must consider all plans (and attempts) based on the intent behind them.

Other Areas to Consider . There are, of course, other areas to consider when assessing students for suicide risk. All of the risk factors, warning signs, and protective factors that were included in Chapters 2 and 3, as well as many others, can help determine risk. Some of the areas that are most often included in risk assessments of children and adolescents are included below. However, these are simply guidelines. Individual risk factors may differ for individual students, and that is the key reason for using assessment interviews to gather information. It is in talking with students and developing rapport that we learn what may be behind their suicidal thoughts and behaviors, regardless of whether they "tick boxes" on these lists of risk factors.

Hopelessness/Psychological Pain

Edwin Schneidman (2005), the father of suicidology, coined the term "psychache" to describe the extreme psychological pain of the suicidal person. The basic formula for a suicidal crisis is "emotional or physical pain that [the person believes] is intolerable, inescapable, and interminable" (Chiles & Strosahl, 2005, p. 63). Remember, our assessment of the student's situation doesn't matter. When we look at the student's problems through adult eyes, it might not seem so bad. But students lack adult perspectives. It is the perception of the student regarding this pain that is important. A risk assessment attempts to understand to what levels the student will go (including death) to avoid the pain or because they cannot imagine that a situation will ever improve. When assessing this psychache, we must understand and acknowledge the emotional desperation and unbearable emotions that the student feels. If the student perceives that we are saying or doing *anything* that diminishes or disconfirms the level of pain they feel or how hopeless they think the situation is, it can lead to escalation. If the pain is not acknowledged, students might think, "You don't understand how bad I really feel. Let me show you."

Practical strategy (schools): Acknowledging the pain and the hopelessness does not mean that you have to agree that the situation is hopeless. It only means that we recognize that the student feels this way. In the next chapter, you will learn some strategies to help instill hope. For now, recognizing the adolescent perspective is key to assessment. To help with this perspective, you might remember a painful breakup you had as an adolescent, only to have an adult tell you, "You're young. You'll find someone else." Perhaps you remember how unhelpful this type of comment was.

History of Suicidal Thoughts or Behaviors/
Suicide Among Family or Friends

A previous suicide attempt has long been considered to be a predictor of future attempts. However, recent research has led us to understand that this may not be true for many adolescents who die by suicide (Franklin et al., 2017). In other words, there are some adolescents who have frequent attempts, and there are some children and adolescents who have one, lethal suicide completion. In short, we are less clear about how suicide attempts factor into deaths than we once were. However, we do know this: Students with a history of suicidal thoughts and behaviors are likely to engage in future suicidal thoughts and behaviors. In addition, students who engage in *any sort of behavioral rehearsal* (e.g., putting a rope around their neck to see how it feels; standing on the edge of a building or bridge, looking down, and imagining jumping; taking out pills and counting them) are at much higher risk for engaging in suicidal behaviors.

As we assess the student's own history of suicidal behaviors, we also consider suicidal behaviors within the family. There is evidence that young people can model these behaviors from other members in the family. They might think, "This is how we handle stressful situations in my family." Recent suicides among their peer group can also serve as models, and there is always concerns about contagion in schools. This can occur in the aftermath of a student suicide or on significant anniversaries.

Mental State/Substance Use/Stability of Mood

Many students who die by suicide have some underlying mental health condition, most often depression, anxiety, or trauma. Others have substance use problems, which can exacerbate the mood condition. Whether or not there is an underlying mental health condition or substance use problem, assessing the current mood state is important. Most often, suicidal students present as hopeless, helpless, impulsive, agitated, stressed, worthless, or consumed by self-hatred. Each of these mood states can play a role in suicide risk.

Warning Signs or Triggering Conditions

Suicide typically doesn't just come out of nowhere. For most students, this isn't just a moment in time, but a trajectory that builds and builds. As conditions deteriorate for the student, they often exhibit more and more warning signs. We discussed many of these in Chapter 3. For example, they might withdraw, express their suicidal thoughts verbally or in writing, give away their prized possessions, and/or seek out means, such as a gun or pills. As they move further along in this trajectory, for some students, something will happen that becomes the proverbial "straw that broke the camel's back." This becomes the triggering condition—something that exceeds their capacity to cope. It can be big or small—but it is simply too much for them to handle. Triggering conditions can be social embarrassment, academic difficulties, bullying or victimization, conflict with friends or family, difficult and unavoidable transitions or circumstances, or countless others. Recognizing the warning signs and triggering conditions can also provide insight into the mind of the suicidal student.

In a tragic story from our own work, a young college woman killed herself on a night that she called her mother to ask if the mother would pick her up from college so she could come home for the weekend. Her mother told her daughter that she already had plans to visit one of her other children at a different university that weekend, but perhaps they could make plans for a different weekend in the future. The young woman killed herself that night. Of course, she didn't kill herself because she couldn't go home that weekend. A psychological autopsy (a look at what was going on in the person's life before the suicide) revealed that she had been spiraling into a severe depression over several months. She was isolating, using substances, not going to classes, and having relationship problems. *All of her friends and peers* knew it, but not one reached out and no one told her family or anyone at the university who could help. The point of this story is that it is easy to look at the triggering event (in this case, a visit home) and make simplistic assumptions.

Another triggering condition occurred at a local private high school. A very successful high school senior was involved in a terrible car accident and found to be under the influence of alcohol. A child in the other car was seriously hurt, and there was a long court case. The young man was publicly shamed, and he began to isolate and withdraw, use more substances, and ultimately had a suicide attempt. Once in counseling, it was clear that he had a long history of severe depression. The car accident was a triggering event for him. Although it was heartbreaking and would have been difficult for *any* young person to manage, his already depleted coping left him unable to face the challenges of the situation.

Protective Factors

Suicide risk assessment also includes protective factors. What are the things within the environment that are helping to keep the student safe? Do they have the support of a caring family or friends? Are they currently receiving treatment, or if they have received treatment in the past, can their individual therapist be contacted for ongoing interventions (with parental involvement and proper releases, of course)? What resources can they identify that can help if they are in crisis? What are the strengths the student can identify? In general, research supports the role of protective factors in reducing future attempts, although there is less clear evidence about its role in protecting against suicide death (Franklin et al., 2017).

Nevertheless, we believe that it is *vital* to include an assessment of protective factors when assessing suicide risk, if only to remind students that they have intrapersonal and interpersonal strengths to rely upon to help them through the crisis.

> *Practical strategy (schools): One way to assess a student's protective factors is through a quick assessment of what is keeping the student alive. Marsha Linehan (1981) developed several Reasons for Living inventories for different age groups, all of which are publicly available, with a quick Internet search. Because these scales are not intended to yield "scores" or answers, they are helpful simply to guide discussion around protective factors during assessment interviews.*

Using an Acronym and Checklists to Guide Assessment Interviews. Sometimes, acronyms can help guide the risk assessment, reminding the interviewer of some of the major areas to cover. These should be used with caution, however, as they are simply reminders of areas to assess and do not provide scores or answers.

The American Association of Suicidology recommends IS PATH WARM? as a helpful mnemonic (Figure 8.1). Each letter corresponds to an important risk factor for suicide. Although other acronyms exist to help with suicide assessment, IS PATH WARM? is the agreed-upon standard acronym for suicide risk assessment, including for guiding assessments within schools (Juhnke et al., 2007).

Specifically, these warning signs are linked to:

- Ideation about suicide, including talking about or writing about suicide or death
- Substance (alcohol or drug) use, particularly increases in use
- Purposelessness, no reason for living, no sense of meaning in life
- Anxiety, agitation, inability to sleep (or sleeping all the time), unable to relax, extreme perturbation

I	Ideation
S	Substance Abuse
P	Purposelessness
A	Anxiety
T	Trapped
H	Hopelessness
W	Withdrawal
A	Anger
R	Recklessness
M	Mood Change

Figure 8.1 IS PATH WARM?
Source: American Association of Suicidology (2006).

- **T**rapped, no way out of the current situation, no other choices between living in extreme psychological pain or death
- **H**opelessness and helplessness, including negative view of self, others, and the future
- **W**ithdrawal from friends, family, and society or activities that used to bring pleasure
- **A**nger, rage, uncontrolled fury, seeking revenge
- **R**eckless behaviors, engaging in risky activities, seemingly without thinking
- **M**ood changes that are dramatic and erratic

There are many checklists that are available to guide questioning around suicide risk. However, just as with the "IS PATH WARM? acronym, these checklists are intended only as a guide for the assessment interview, not as a definitive suicide risk assessment. They are useful to the degree to which they help us remember the important areas to cover. Sometimes we talk with school personnel who worry that during the middle of talking to a potentially suicidal student, they might forget some of the major areas to cover. They are concerned that their own anxieties will get in the way. In these instances, a checklist might be useful, but only to help guide the process. Two cautions are necessary. First, if students perceive you are just "reading questions off of a standard checklist," it may have negative consequences for rapport. Be careful about stilted or "canned" approaches to a suicide risk assessment interview. Second, some suicide risk checklists include "objective" scoring systems that yield a number at the end that is then linked to a predetermined level of suicide risk. These scoring systems are *extremely dangerous* and can encourage inappropriate use. We recommend removing all scoring from any checklist that is used and keeping the questions and/or topics covered as *general guidelines only*. We also are very careful not to categorize students into low/medium/high risk. These categories can lead to simplistic assumptions and generalized interventions. Suicide risk assessment is more complicated than scores or risk levels can make us believe.

Typical questions on a suicide assessment checklist typically include these areas (not necessarily in this order and not limited to just these questions):

- Questions about suicidal thoughts
  - o Does the student have frequent suicidal thoughts?
  - o When did the thoughts first occur?
  - o What led up to the thoughts?
  - o How close have they come to acting on these thoughts?
  - o Are these thoughts intrusive and/or out of the student's control?
  - o Does the student believe they are likely to act on these suicidal thoughts?
  - o Has the student spoken to anyone else about the suicidal thoughts?
- Questions about suicidal behaviors
  - o Has the student had a suicide attempt in the past?

- o Does the student have a detailed plan?
- o Does the student have access to the means to complete the plan?
- o Has the student made any arrangements to complete the plan?
- o Has the student engaged in behavioral rehearsal (started to act out the plan)?
- Questions about state of mind
  - o Is the student in severe psychological distress?
  - o Does the student feel hopeless?
  - o Is the student demonstrating changes in mood?
  - o Does the student display poor impulse control?
  - o Does the student have cognitive rigidity/poor problem-solving?
  - o Does the student fantasize about death or the afterlife?
- Questions about behaviors
  - o Is the student demonstrating changes in behavior?
  - o Is the student isolating or withdrawing?
  - o Is the student actively using substances?
- Questions about environment
  - o Does the student have any recent, severe stressors?
  - o Is there a history of family violence?
  - o Is there a history of or current trauma or abuse?
- Questions about recent events
  - o Is there a triggering event that is escalating the student?
  - o Is the student demonstrating warning signs such as the following:
    - Talking or writing about suicide
    - Doing Internet searches about death or suicide
    - Giving away prized possessions
    - Obtaining the means to complete suicide
    - Making final arrangements
    - Engaging in increased risk-taking
- Questions about protective factors

- o Does the student have a strong support system?
- o Does the student have a trusted adult to talk with about suicidal thoughts?
- o Can the student identify any reasons for living?

In general, using a checklist can help a school-based suicide risk assessor cover the major areas that should be included in the assessment. These checklist questions also can serve as a springboard for further discussion and exploration of important topics. Finally, checklists can be useful for documentation purposes.

Formal (Standardized) Assessments. There are dozens of published standardized suicide risk assessments and hundreds of unpublished questionnaires and assessments available for use. There is, however, great variability in their quality, and some published instruments have very low reliability and validity. Those that are well established and have sound psychometric properties are copyrighted and must be purchased. Therefore, we cannot share them with you here, other than to tell you that the Substance Abuse and Mental Health Services Administration is working to keep a list of psychometrically sound assessments on their website (https://www.samhsa.gov/suicide). Standardized assessments can be useful in providing adjunctive information that helps get a clearer picture of the situation, but they are seldom used in schools.

Some Final Thoughts on Assessment Interviews. We know that assessment of suicide risk is complicated, and we have provided a lot of information. We return to the start of this section, which is that the most important thing you can do is to *ask the question* and open the conversation. Once you have, you will be asked to make a determination about what to do next. Clearly, this will involve informing parents. When you do, you will want to give them *as much information as possible* so they can make informed decisions. This is why your initial discussions with the student should be clear, follow a predetermined developmentally appropriate protocol, and be documented. Before you engage in your school-based initial risk assessment, we offer these overall thoughts to help guide you through the process (Granello, 2010).

- **Assessment of each person is unique.**

Part of the difficulty in assessing suicide risk is that there have been over 100 risk factors that have been identified in the research. Assessing the known risk factors is helpful because, in general, the more risk factors a person has, the higher their risk. *However,* all of these risk factors are based on population-based data and long-term outcomes. They simply don't tell us as much as we would like about an individual student's short-term risk. That is the benefit of the assessment interview. It allows the student's story to be heard, with emphasis on the risks, and protective factors, for that specific person.

- **Assessment is complex and challenging.**

Most people who are suicidal are ambivalent. They don't want to die. They simply want the pain to go away. That means that the person may not know whether or not they actually intend to die. As a result, the person doing the assessment is trying to measure something that *even the student being assessed doesn't know the answer to.* That makes suicide risk assessment different from almost anything else that we assess, and it adds to the complexity.

- **Assessment is an ongoing process.**

Suicide risk can change quickly. Students who are at slightly elevated risk one day can move to much higher risk the next. This is true for all suicidal people, but even more of a problem for children and adolescents, where impulsivity is more likely to play a role in suicide than it does for adults. Frequent check-ins and ongoing assessments are a must for all students who have any risk for suicide.

- **Assessment errs on the side of caution.**

This may seem obvious. When in doubt, we always assume higher risk. There simply are no second chances.

- **Assessment is collaborative.**

Multiple perspective provide the best suicide risk assessments. The Family Educational Rights and Privacy Act (FERPA) and the Health Insurance Portability and Accountability Act (HIPPA) both have exceptions for safety of the child. This does not mean that everyone in the school needs to know everything about a student's suicide risk, but it does mean that if there are staff, teachers, or students with information that will help, then that information is discreetly and carefully collected. Remember, suicide risk assessments are collaborative (done with other professionals), corroborative (done with information from anyone who can provide it), and consultative (done with supervision and support).

- **Assessment relies on clinical judgment.**

Ultimately, there is no checklist or assessment that will provide a definitive answer about a student's suicide risk. Once all the information is collected, someone at the school will need to decide what happens next, and of course, that will involve parents. With training, supervision, and experience, the initial suicide risk assessments that are done in schools can become less overwhelming, but it is always a difficult task. Data and information collected from the student and others during risk assessment can help ensure that these initial judgments have a solid grounding.

- **Assessment takes all threats, warning signs, and risk factors seriously.**

Most students demonstrate clear warning signs, and in fact, tell other people, before they have a suicide attempt or completion. However, for many students, either these warning signs are not recognized for what they are or the messages they tell others are never repeated to adults who know what to do.

- **Assessment asks the tough questions.**

Sometimes, when students are suicidal, they speak in euphemisms (e.g., "They won't have me to kick around anymore" or "They'll be sorry"). But when it comes to suicide risk assessment, it is important to be *very clear, very precise, and to use the word "suicide."*

- **Assessment is intervention.**

Mental health professionals know that the telling of the story is, in and of itself, curative. Feeling heard and understood is powerful, and the rapport that is developed through the initial suicide assessment interview can make students feel valued, respected, and cared for. Although this is not sufficient for healing, it certainly starts the student on a path toward healing.

- **Assessment tries to uncover the underlying message.**

As the student tells the story of their suicide risk, astute mental health professionals listen for why the student is suicidal. For example, the student might be using the suicide (or attempt) to *communicate* something, to *control* the behavior of others, or to *avoid* something. Once the underlying message is clear, this information can be used to help with intervention.

- **Assessment is done in a cultural context.**

Allowing students to talk about suicide, including their own thoughts, feelings, and risk and protective factors, in ways and words that are most comfortable is important (with the caveat that the word "suicide" is part of this conversation).

- **Assessment is documented.**

Schools are legally required to document suicide risk assessment. Documenting the process helps make sure that protocols were followed. It also helps school systems reflect on, and learn from, the process.

Conclusion

Students who are at risk for suicide need special attention in schools. Selective interventions are for students who have certain risk factors that require remediation and support. When these students are identified, helping them connect to selective interventions means that they can receive school-based interventions that help them develop positive social and emotional skills. Indicated interventions are for those students who have been identified as at risk for suicide. These students must first be identified through a prompt and accurate school-based suicide risk assessment. School-based risk assessments are not the same as comprehensive suicide risk assessments, but they typically are conducted with a semistructured interview that guides the assessor and student through major areas of risk so that information can be shared with parents and treating professionals.

References

American Association of Suicidology. (2006). *Warning signs for suicide.* http://www.suicidology.org/web/guest/stats-and-tools/warning-signs

American Foundation for Suicide Prevention, American School Counselor Association, National Association of School Psychologists & The Trevor Project (2019). *Model School District Policy on Suicide Prevention: Model Language, Commentary, and Resources* (2nd ed.). New York: American Foundation for Suicide Prevention.

American School Counselor Association. (2020). *The school counselor and suicide risk assessment.* https://www.schoolcounselor.org/

Byars, J., Graybill, E., Wellons, Q., & Harper, L. (2020). Monitoring social media and technology use to prevent youth suicide and school violence. *Contemporary School Psychology, 24,* 318–326.

Chiles, J. A., & Strosahl, K. D. (2005). *Clinical manual for assessment and treatment of suicidal patients.* American Psychiatric Association.

Cvek, V. (2017). Policing social media: Balancing the interests of schools and students and providing universal protection for students' rights. *Penn State Law Review, 121*(2), 583–616.

Czeisler, M. E., Lane, R. I., Petrosky, E., Wiley, J. F., Christensen, A., Njai, R., Weaver, M. D., Robbins, R., Facer-Childs, E. R., Barger, L. K., Czeisler, C. A., Howard, M. E., & Rajaratnam, S. M. W. (2020). Mental health, substance use, and suicidal ideation during the COVID-19 pandemic—United States, June 24–30, 2020. *MMWR Morbidity Mortality Weekly Report, 69,* 1049–1057. doi:10.15585/mmwr.mm6932a1external icon

Erbacher, T. A., Singer, J. B., & Poland, S. (2015). *Suicide in schools: A practitioner's guide to multi-level prevention, assessment, intervention, and postvention.* Routledge.

Franklin, J. C., Ribeiro, J. D., Fox, K. R., Bentley, K. H., Kleiman, E. M., Huang, X., Musacchio, K. M., Jaroszewski, A. C., Chang, B. P., & Nock, M. K. (2017). Risk factors for suicidal thoughts and behaviors: A meta-analysis of 50 years of research. *Psychological Bulletin, 143*(2), 187–232.

Granello, D. H. (2010). The process of suicide risk assessment: Twelve core principles. *Journal of Counseling & Development, 88,* 363–371.

Juhnke, G. A., Granello, P. F., & Lebrón-Striker, M. A. (2007). *IS PATH WARM? A suicide assessment mnemonic for counselors (ACAPCD-03).* American Counseling Association.

Linehan, M. (1981). *Suicidal behaviors questionnaire.* Unpublished inventory. University of Washington, Seattle, Washington.

McGlothlin, J. (2008). *Developing clinical skills in suicide assessment, prevention and treatment.* American Counseling Association

National Association of School Psychologists. (2019). *Preventing suicide: Guidelines for administrators and crisis teams.* https://www.nasponl ine.org

Rogers, C. R. (1957). The necessary and sufficient conditions of therapeutic personality change. *Journal of Consulting Psychology, 21,* 95–103.

Shneidman, E. S. (2005). How I read. *Suicide and Life-Threatening Behavior, 35*(2), 117–120.

9

Working With Suicidal Students in Schools

Intervention

In the previous chapter, we discussed how to identify specific students who might be at risk for suicide. In this chapter, we move directly to intervention. Notice that we do not frame this as treatment. Schools are *not* the place to engage in the clinical treatment of suicidal students. Rather, quality school-based suicide prevention programs should detect students who are at risk for suicide, conduct basic risk assessments, and help refer students to competent care.

In general, there are three types of students who will require school-based suicide interventions. First, there are students who are chronically suicidal. These students go through periods of time (days, weeks, or months) with low-level chronic suicide ideation. They may escalate to higher suicide risk and require ongoing monitoring and support. The second type of student is the one who is in some type of suicide crisis. These are students who come to the attention of school-based mental health professionals, who are assessed for suicidality, and who require additional assessment or referral. The third type of student is the one who is returning to school following some type of suicide crisis or inpatient mental health treatment. Each of these students will need individualized attention with a well-thought-through approach for how the school can support the student without encouraging contagion, overstepping the boundaries of the school staff, or inappropriately

Suicide and Self-Injury in Schools. Darcy Haag Granello, Paul F. Granello, Gerald A. Juhnke, Oxford University Press. © Oxford University Press 2023. DOI: 10.1093/oso/9780190059842.003.0009

disrupting the school environment. Before we turn our attention to strategies to help these students, let's first turn to a general overview of school-based suicide intervention.

School-Based Intervention Tasks

Because the goal of the school is *not* to provide clinical interventions but instead to facilitate local referrals, one of the most important first steps is to identify a network of local mental health providers to whom students can be referred. School mental health professionals should reach out to these providers to develop positive and strong working relationships so that when crises arise, they are knowledgeable about the services they offer, the types of clients they see, the insurance plans they accept, and the sliding fee scale they offer (if any). The Substance Abuse and Mental Health Services Administration (SAMHSA; 2012) provides a list of the types of local service providers to whom students might be referred. Some examples of providers include:

- Hospitals, especially emergency departments (or pediatric hospitals, if available)
- Psychiatric hospitals
- Community mental health centers
- Individual mental health providers (e.g., child psychiatrists, psychologists, counselors, and/or social workers)
- Primary care providers
- Spiritual leaders and/or traditional healers

A second task to accomplish *before* there is a crisis is to develop all the necessary forms that will be required during suicide intervention. Providers might be able to assist schools as they develop appropriate protocols and paperwork for referrals. For example, schools will need documentation paperwork for assessment, forms indicating when parents/guardians were notified and by whom, the types of community referrals that were made, and release of information forms for community providers, among others. All of these forms should be completed and compiled in an easy-to-find location. Staff who will need to use the forms will require training on them, including how to handle confidentiality requirements.

Finally, prior to the implementation of any suicide intervention, there must be guidelines for how to notify parents or guardians of a student's suicide risk. There is clear consensus among the major school-based mental health professions (e.g., counselors, school psychologists, social workers) that a student's legal guardians should be notified in the case of a student's suicide ideation or behaviors. Having clear guidelines and talking points is helpful to ensure these conversations are calm and professional.

> *Practical strategy (schools): Everything that occurs around suicide assessment and intervention should be documented. This includes signed acknowledgment from parents/guardians that they have been notified by the school about the student's suicide risk. SAMHSA (2012) has a free toolkit for schools that has examples of many of the forms that are required or recommended for schools to use during suicide intervention.*

Interventions With Suicidal Students

In the following sections, we will discuss strategies for working with students during these three major times that they present as suicidal in the school building. These include students who are chronically suicidal, students who are in suicidal crisis, and those who return to the school building after they have been hospitalized or in some type of mental health care that has removed them from the school environment.

Chronically Suicidal Students

In any school, there are students who are chronically suicidal. The reasons for the chronic suicidality of these students may range from specific mental health conditions (depression, anxiety, emerging personality disorders) to early childhood trauma (attachment disorders, physical or emotional abuse) or even chronic adverse environmental conditions (poverty, bullying, systemic racism). Chances are, it is a combination of factors that contributes to each student's risk. Regardless of the reason(s), students who have on-going suicidal ideation can occupy a lot of time and resources. Moreover, because of the chronicity of their distress, they can be emotionally draining on those around them, including school-based mental health professionals.

Often these students have strong feelings of worthlessness and hopelessness. Younger students may have more somatic complaints such as headaches or muscle tension. They may frequently be sent to the nurse's or counselor's office by concerned teachers or peers. In any school building we enter, there are students who are well known to the administrators and mental health professionals in the building because of their ongoing distress. These students may talk about, write about, and think about suicide. They are often self-referred. Yet, these students are not currently suicidal. That is, they do not have an active plan or intent. For them, suicide is a *possibility* that they are not willing to take off the table. Chronically suicidal students are in pain, and they walk around the school building each day knowing that suicide is an option that they may use in the future.

Practical strategy (schools and parents): Chronically suicidal students talk about suicide so often that staff may begin to become habituated to their words and stop taking them seriously. We hear it all the time ("Oh, she's always threatening suicide!"). This is very dangerous. We can never ignore a student's talk of suicide. When we do, we force them to escalate. The best way to explain this is through an example.

We once worked with the mother of a 7-year-old, who said her daughter "threatened suicide" whenever she was upset. Our response was, that wasn't how she first tried to get her mother's attention. A long time ago, when she wanted her mother's attention, she did or said something less dramatic. When that stopped working, she escalated. She continued escalating her words and threats until she found herself having to "threaten" suicide to get her mother's attention. Once that stops working, she has no place to go except to escalate to behaviors (suicide attempts).

The same is true in schools. Students who "threaten" suicide to "get attention" need attention. That is clear. If we refuse to give them attention, they have no recourse but to escalate to higher levels to get our attention. We force them into it. When we hear staff say things like "She's just doing it to get attention," our response is, "Then give her some attention!" Then, when the student (or daughter) is _not_ in crisis, teach them how to get our attention is _appropriate_ ways. Finally (and this is the hard part), when they do the thing that we taught them and seek our attention in appropriate ways, we have to give them our attention. We might give them our attention in weekly check-ins or groups. We also might give them our attention when they seek us out with appropriate statements, telling us that they need help. We _guarantee_ that they will do this at the most inconvenient times! It _always_ seems to work like that! Whether it is intentional or not, it seems that when we teach people how to seek our attention appropriately, they seem to "test it out" at 5:00 when we have dinner guests on the way over or when we have other commitments on our time. Nevertheless, we have to drop what we are doing and give our students, our children, or our clients, attention. (After all, our dinner guests are adults. They know what we do for a living. They will keep themselves entertained for 15 minutes while we reinforce these important new behaviors in our students or clients.)

Students who are chronically suicidal can represent a challenge from a suicide intervention standpoint. On suicide risk assessments, they do not reach the level of needing immediate care. Nevertheless, they cannot be deemed "no risk" either. They are, quite simply, in an ongoing, low-risk category. In all cases, it is important to notify the parents of these students early on for a comprehensive suicide risk assessment and for an external mental health referral. This is important, because *always* when schools conduct a suicide risk assessment *of any type* with students, regardless of outcome, parents must be notified. But for the students in this category, the risk of suicide is not imminent, and the mental health struggles continue, with suicide always a potential future outcome.

Practical strategy (schools): One strategy to help students who are chronically suicidal is with a monitoring routine. In coordination with an outside referral (if appropriate, and if releases have been signed), these students can be assessed periodically for increases in suicidal ideation or thoughts of self-harm. In addition, the amount of school-based services provided to a student can be adjusted to increase in times of need or tapered when the student is doing better. Data on baseline behavior can be charted and used as a comparison point. Finally, scheduling regular appointments or including the student in a weekly group can help reduce the student's perceived need to just drop by the nurse's station or the counseling office.

Students in Suicide Crisis

When students have been assessed for suicide and determined to be at risk (see Chapter 8), a clear protocol will guide the next steps in the process. Involving parents in the development of these policies can help ensure that they are written in a way that promotes positive interactions between school personnel and parents. There is evidence that schools that have active and involved parents in the development of policies and procedures that relate to the health of their students are more likely to have successful outcomes when parents need to be involved (Centers for Disease Control and Prevention, 2012).

Working With Parents . Once the imminent safety of the student is assured, the parents or legal guardians must be notified. This holds true unless it is clear that the parents or guardians will escalate the suicide risk (or in cases of abuse), in which case Child Protective Services (CPS) should be called. In all cases, it is important that the legal guardians (and we will use the term "parents," with the recognition that it may be guardians or CPS) should be given as much information as possible about what the school has learned about the student's potential risk (that is the "corroboration" part of risk assessment). This includes the results of any school-based risk assessment, any verbal or written indications that the student has made of suicide, or any other information that has come to the attention of the mental health professionals who have conducted the school-based assessment. *This is important* so that anyone conducting a risk assessment at the next level has all the information to help determine the student's risk.

We recognize that notifying a parent that their child is at risk for suicide can be challenging, to say the least. Parents can have a wide range of responses, and school mental health professionals must be prepared to manage those responses. The ultimate goal is that schools and parents work together to keep the student safe and to get them the care they need. Parents might welcome this assistance from the school. They might also feel threatened or confused. They may also be in denial about the level of distress their child is in. Whatever the parents' response, it is important to stay focused and clear, to give parents all of the information available that led to the concerns about the student's risk, and to strongly encourage parents to seek additional mental health care for their child (American School Counselor Association, 2020).

Practical strategy (schools): In Chapter 5, when we spoke about reaching out parents to discuss a student's nonsuicidal self-injury behaviors, we offered some practical strategies for how to partner with parents who may have difficulty processing what they are learning about their child's behavior. Those strategies apply for potentially suicidal students as well, and we encourage you to read those strategies so you can apply them to this situation (p. XX). We also believe it is important to help parents understand the next steps in the process as students go through a suicide risk assessment and possibly a referral for a more intensive level of care. This can be a scary time for parents, and we have learned that at least part of their negative emotional reaction can be based simply on the fear of not knowing what comes next. They may even have some faulty assumptions or stories about counseling or psychiatric care based on the entertainment industry or stories on social media. A calm, reasonable discussion that informs parents of what options are available, what will happen when they take their child to the different places on the referral list, and what assessment and referral will look like can help allay some of those fears.

After a school notifies a parent or legal guardian of a student's risk for suicide and provides referral information, the responsibility to seek mental health assistance for the child falls on the parent. In most cases, *only* if the student is in a suicide emergency (e.g., imminent threat, such as having a gun or knife or standing on a ledge) can the school require that the student be transported to emergency mental health care. This underscores the importance of helping parents become partners with the school in intervention, rather than see the school as threatening or invasive. In all cases, schools should know their local laws and district policies regarding the decisions about transporting students without parental consent *before* a crisis occurs.

Practical strategy (parents): When students have any elevated risk for suicide, parents should remove means from the household. In fact, means restriction is one of the most important strategies for suicide prevention. Means restriction works because for many youth, suicide crises are short term, so reducing access to means during those crises can help save lives. For most young people, the average amount of time between when they decide to kill themselves and when they have an attempt is less than 10 minutes. That means that anything that can be done to interrupt their behaviors and increase the amount of time between the young person's decision to die by suicide and their access to means has the potential to help. Although some youth might select another method for suicide if their first option is unavailable, research consistently finds that many do not (Giggie et al., 2007). Families who are given education and information about means restriction are more likely to take these important steps to save the lives of their children. For more information, visit the Means Matter website at https://www.hsph.harvard.edu/means-matter/.

Practical strategy (schools): As school-based mental health professionals educate parents and families about ways to help them sanitize the environment, we have learned that how this is framed is important. For example, asking families to "get rid of" their guns may not be helpful. Rather, asking if they would be willing to have guns stored at another location—perhaps at the home of a relative or trusted friend—until the suicide crisis has been resolved is often much more productive.

In all cases, parents should sign a standardized form indicating that they understand that their child is at risk for suicide and that the school has provided resources and referrals. In cases where a specific referral is made and a parent agrees (and signs a release), it may be possible for a school to send information directly to an outside referral agency. *However*, doing so may also place a financial obligation on the school for the care of the student. Therefore, in general, the school's obligation is to give information about referrals as well as specific information about the student's risk directly to the parent or legal guardian.

Working With Outside Providers . Most students who are assessed for suicide risk by an outside provider will engage in some type of outpatient therapy. These students will remain in the school, perhaps missing only an afternoon or a day of school as they are assessed and linked to services. In these cases, it is the responsibility of the school mental health professionals to support the primarily therapeutic interventions the student is receiving in outpatient care. Of course, this can only be done if the proper releases are signed and if the parent, student, and external provider agree that the school can and should function in this role. Importantly, this does *not* mean that the school should provide a therapeutic intervention. It only means that the school system should, when possible, support the development and maintenance of behaviors and skills that are being developed in the student's outpatient counseling.

In general, several types of outpatient therapeutic interventions have been found to be effective with suicidal young people (Singer et al., 2017). Of course, individual practitioners or agencies may use different approaches in their work, but these are the overarching approaches that have the most research effectiveness behind them. We offer them only as general guidelines to support healthy interactions with suicidal students. We *do not believe it is appropriate* for school-based mental health professionals to offer this type of intervention for suicidal students within the context of the school setting. Further, it is important that school-based professionals *not attempt to engage in intensive therapy* with suicidal students without first understanding the type of treatment the student is receiving from an off-campus provider. The ethical codes of all the helping professions clearly state that treating professionals *should not* attempt to engage in therapy with anyone who is under the clinical care of another professional. It is important to keep these boundaries clear.

- **Attachment-based family therapy**. This type of therapy is effective because it includes family members, and suicide in young people has been linked to interactional patterns in families. Interrupting those patterns has been shown to reduce suicide ideation. This is primarily done through reframing the adolescent's suicide risk as a relational issue rather than an individual one, as well as helping the adolescent attach to the parent in healthy ways. These strategies are intended to help the young person feel secure, safe, and protected within the family unit (Diamond, 2014).
- **Integrated cognitive behavioral therapy**. This therapy uses social cognitive learning theory to help young people identify and reframe maladaptive thoughts about themselves and others and to learn new social skills. This is primarily done through learning how to develop intentional strategies for making decisions and how to set appropriate goals, using techniques that are often used in motivational interviewing (W. R. Miller & Rollnick, 2013).
- **Dialectical behavior therapy for adolescents**. Adapted from Linehan's dialectical behavior therapy (DBT; Linehan, 1993), this therapy teaches adolescents how to tolerate negative emotions while simultaneously developing strategies for change. Techniques such as emotion regulation, distress tolerance, and behavioral (chain) analysis are all part of this approach (A. L. Miller et al., 2007).

There are many specific strategies that schools can use to help support students who are struggling with suicidal thoughts and behaviors while they are getting assistance from outside resources. Many of these strategies are the same, whether the student is remaining in school or returning to school after spending time in an inpatient unit. Therefore, rather than repeat them in both sections, we have consolidated them all below.

Students Returning School After a Suicide Crisis

Planning for a student's safe return to school following a suicide crisis can help protect the individual student involved as well as limit the potential for contagion to other students. Remember the student may be behind in their academic work, may continue to be overwhelmed by the enormity of the situation, and may be taking medications that interfere with their ability to do their work. These considerations, and others, require clear planning and preparation so that schools can provide the most supportive, and least restrictive, environment for the student to thrive. In this section, we will discuss some overall protocols that may be helpful as well as specific strategies and interventions that we have found to be useful. Again, the goal is *not* to provide suicide-specific interventions, but rather to support the mental health treatment that is occurring outside of the school building.

Following a Standardized Protocol. Just as with the suicide risk assessment and the initial interactions with parents when a student is at risk for suicide, having clear protocols in place for when students return to school after they have been away receiving crisis support and treatment helps everyone in the school know how to best respond. Each step in the process is designed to provide structure, safety, and support.

Sadly, many students who are involved in some type of crisis support (typically hospitalization or inpatient care) return to school having received very little in the way of therapy, education, or mood stabilization. In fact, whereas students in suicide crisis were once sent to residential facilities to receive ongoing care, the reality of today's treatment environments is that many students who receive inpatient care often do not even have time to stabilize on medication before they are discharged. Therefore, when they return to school, it is possible, maybe even probable, that very little has fundamentally changed since the moment they were taken out of school, oftentimes just days prior. It is for this reason that many suicidologists question whether inpatient treatment, once considered the "gold standard" of care, is always the best option for suicidal youth. Regardless of the decision to hospitalize youth (a decision that is typically not made by school staff), the reality is that when students return to school, many will still have high levels of distress.

Hold a Re-entry Meeting.   Before the student is allowed back in the school building, there should be an in-person meeting with everyone who will be involved with the student's case. At a minimum, this means the school counselor (or other mental health professional who will be overseeing the student's case), school nurse (if available, particularly if the student is on medication), school-based social worker or other case manager, school administrator(s) who will be involved with the student's case, student, and parent(s)/legal guardian(s).

By the end of the re-entry meeting, everyone involved should understand the following:

- The specific needs of the student, including the specific strategies each member of the team should use to help support the student
- The safety plan, as outlined in the discharge paperwork, and the role of each team member in facilitating that safety plan (as appropriate to share with team members)
- The medication support that is needed for the student
- The clear expectations of the student (academic, behavioral, attendance, etc.)
- The future expectations of all parties (including how to let others know if any of the expectations change)
- The message that is to be given to teachers about expectations (Remember that although teachers *should not be informed about the details of the student's mental health situation*, they will need to know what accommodations are expected of them.)
- The date for follow-up

Even before the re-entry meeting, it is wise to consider any potential barriers that could limit the effectiveness of the student's re-entry. In our experience, we have found that parents might be reluctant to share information (including discharge paperwork and safety plans) from outside providers, sometimes because they have shared information with school systems before, with bad outcomes (or have heard stories from other parents about negative experiences). We have also heard from parents that during these re-entry meetings, they have felt pressured by school administrators or nurses to increase a student's medication. However, it is not, of course, the role of the school to give advice about medication. As a result, parents may come to re-entry meetings perceiving the school as an adversary. School personnel might also join these meetings feeling frustrated, believing that they are simply trying to help the student and perceiving that the parents are thwarting their attempts. In short, there can be a lot of unspoken messages that make these re-entry meetings difficult. The more that school mental health professionals use their interpersonal skills to clear the air and work to form an alliance on behalf of the student, the better the chances of a productive meeting.

Practical strategy (schools): Because parents are often concerned about what has happened in the past (even if the information is "true"—or simply rumors from other parents), they may be reluctant to share information in the re-entry meeting, which can greatly reduce the school's ability to develop a productive strategy for the student. We have found that helping the parents have a sense of control can be very useful. Simple strategies, such as setting (and keeping) clear boundaries with the parents about what information will be shared (and with whom), goes a long way. If possible, give parents edit power over what information will be shared with others by allowing them to screen any emails that will go out to teachers and staff. This simple strategy allows parents to feel like they are partners in their child's care.

Practical strategy (schools): Students do not owe anyone any explanation of why they were away from school. Teachers and peers do not need to know what is happening or what is the state of their current mental health. <u>Nevertheless,</u> we know that rumor mills are rampant, and when students return to school, they are often met with curious friends who ask lots of prying questions. We always think it is best to prepare students for what they will say when people confront them about the situation. We remind them that they don't have to say anything about their specific situation, but giving them a chance to write down and <u>practice</u> their responses helps them feel prepared. We have a simple worksheet that prepares students for what they might do or say when they are met with questions from peers, when they need to interact with teachers about missed schoolwork, or when they are faced with teasing or inappropriate online messages. It asks them to think about the following:

- *I want to talk with (e.g., specific teachers/coaches/club leaders)...*
- *I need to talk with this person about...*
- *I have concerns about talking with this person because...*
- *This is what I am going to say/do...*
- *If friends ask me why I was away from school, I will say...*
- *If I am confronted online, I will...*

In other words, the more prepared the student is to face all the possible encounters of life back at school, the more prepared they will be for successful re-entry.

Consider Giving Students a Sense of Control. Students who are returning to school need to know what to do if they become overwhelmed or upset during school hours. It is unfortunate that being in therapy teaches so many emotional regulation skills to young people in distress, and then the school environment doesn't allow them to use these skills when they feel themselves beginning to escalate. Of course, we understand *why* this happens. Schools must provide structure. In the case of suicidal youth, however, it can be counterproductive. We spend so much time in therapy teaching them de-escalation skills but then don't let them use these skills when they need them.

Recently, we did some work at a school with a student in distress who needed to step away from a difficult classroom situation. She asked to use the restroom, because she could feel herself becoming flooded with anxiety and shame when she was working in a small group activity. She was convinced that her classmates were whispering about her and her recent suicidal crisis. When she asked the teacher for a hall pass for the restroom, he handed it to her— attached to the end of a toilet seat. She was mortified and opted not to leave the room at all. Needless to say, she left school that day and did not return. Instead, she ended up back in the inpatient setting. She perceived that school was simply too dangerous of an environment for her, and she saw no reasonable means of escape when she needed to calm herself down.

Practical strategy (schools): Finding a school-wide approach to allowing identified suicidal students a way to calm themselves can be a useful tactic. As an example, we offer the following story, not because we think that this is the exact strategy that every school should use, but because it demonstrates the type of strategy a school might use to help give students a sense of control.

One day, when working with a returning suicidal student, I brought in a "Get out of jail free!" card from my Monopoly set at home. I had been thinking about her return to school, and I knew she was particularly nervous. I considered this student to be at high risk for another suicide attempt. When I saw her the next morning, I handed her the card. I told her, "If you ever feel stressed and overwhelmed and you just can't stay where you are for another moment, you can use this card and come down here to the office. No questions asked." She was incredulous. She asked, "You mean anytime?" "Yes," I said. "Anytime." I explained to her that I trusted her with her own mental health. She had been through a lot, and she knew, better than any of us, what she needed.

I knew this was important for her to have to use in the moment. I didn't want her to have to explain to a teacher that she needed a break. I didn't want her to have to raise her hand and ask permission to take care of herself (and I certainly wouldn't want her to have to carry a restroom key on a toilet seat down the hall). When I gave her the card, I showed her I trusted her and that I thought she was responsible.

Of course, I had to clear it with the administrators and inform all the teachers before I gave the card to her. Several teachers expressed concern. What if, for example, she used the card to get out of a test? What if she skipped an important class? I knew those were potential risks, but the reality was that this was a student at high risk for death. Given that, skipping a class or a test didn't seem too serious.

That student, however, taught me an important lesson that I still remember. She didn't misuse the card. She carried it with her every day, until it started to crumble and turn to dust. In fact, I had to take another card out of my Monopoly set to give to her. This time I had it laminated. In all the months she carried it, she only used the card once. She flashed it to a teacher and came down to my office. I offered her a seat and told her we could talk or she could just sit quietly. She sat for a moment and said, "I'm ready to go back to class now." She didn't need anything. She just wanted to test the system. It worked, she was satisfied, and she never used it again. But she carried the card with her every day, as her own version of a security blanket. She knew that if she needed to, she could escape. Just knowing that was all she needed.

Many schools have similar options. They have quiet rooms, de-escalation passes, and other strategies that allow students to step out when they feel overwhelmed. To use an option like this for students in the building, here are some quick reminders:

- The pass doesn't allow a student to go anywhere, or to go home, take a nap, or go do something fun. It is a specific pass to a specific location.

- Teachers (and everyone in the building) need to be on board. We have heard from too many students that when they try to use their passes, teachers say things like "Okay, you can leave, but just wait 5 more minutes until after I finish explaining this one more thing—it is important." Or they say to the student, "Okay, you can go," but then they roll their eyes. Students see those eyerolls, and they know what that means. They tell us that is why they choose not to leave the room, allowing their emotional dysregulation to escalate. They feel judged for using the pass that is given to them for their safety. If the passes are used, then everyone will need training on how to help students use them effectively.
- It might be helpful to brainstorm with a student five options ahead of time—five different things they can do/places they can go using the pass. The student should decide—and then track how useful and helpful that option was for them on that day. Over time, the student will learn what works for them (and it might be that the entire school might learn what is effective for that school).
- The point of the pass is to "step out"—but what is important (and often missing in these strategies) is to teach students how to "step back in." What do they do/how do they know when they are ready to return to class?

The point is that if we want students to take responsibility for their own mental health, then we have to help them. Clearly, this intervention isn't appropriate for everyone, and certainly there are students who would misuse the privilege. But, at least for some students, it is an important strategy for reintegration into school.

Assign Someone to Help Monitor the Student. Within the school building, identify a person who will help the student readjust to the school environment. This person should check in with the student every day, at least until they have settled back into the school environment, when these check-ins can become less frequent. We have found that there are probably two different people needed here. One is a school mental health professional. This person monitors the student's progress. They ask developmentally appropriate questions, such as how the student is doing, what is their current suicide risk, what is the level of hopelessness, etc. This "mini-assessment" lets the student know that there is a person who is looking out for their mental health. Again, with proper releases signed, the mental health professional in the building will keep an open line of communication with parents and off-campus providers.

Practical strategy (schools): The second person in the school building who assists with the monitoring of the student may be a little less expected. We always ask the student to help us identify a person in the building who they will "eyeball" every day. This person is not a mental health professional, but someone the student identifies as someone they trust and care about. For younger students, it might be their teacher. Older students might identify a teacher, staff member, or coach. Once the staff member is identified, we clear it with the adult to make sure they are okay with this strategy. The point is, the student and adult make brief (just a few seconds) contact every day. Sometimes this is as simple as a "high five" or a quick conversation, but it is every day. If the student doesn't reach out, the staff member looks for the student or contacts the counselor (or administrator) to let them know the contact hasn't occurred. The benefit of this brief encounter is that the student believes they have an ally in the school who cares about them, who notices if they are present, and who seeks them out. This means a lot to students who feel disenfranchised. Students sometimes tell us that mental health professionals "have" to care about them, but they are particularly grateful for the attention they receive from these other staff members. It is just one more way to help them feel connected.

Use a Safety Plan.   Safety plans allow students and school personnel (and others, as appropriate) to develop a concrete, detailed plan that helps the student manage difficult moments or escalating feelings while they are in the school building. The goal of the safety plan, within the school context, is to give the student positive steps that they can complete if they start to feel agitated, upset, hopeless, or helpless. The safety plan reminds them of the coping strategies and resources that they have, both internal and external, and the action steps that they can complete, in sequential order, to help them manage these feelings. The point is, when students are beginning to escalate, they should have a very clear map of how they will manage the situation that they have thought through, with the help of a mental health professional. It is inappropriate and unrealistic to think that students will think on their feet and remember their coping strategies and ideas for managing the situation as the crisis is occurring. Rather, it should all be laid out ahead of time in an easy-to-follow plan.

When working with school-aged youth, safety plans are typically developed by an off-site clinical mental health professional. The role of the school personnel is to be a resource and support mechanism for the student's plan.

Schools should use safety plans instead of "no-suicide contracts" (Chiles & Strosahl, 2005). School professionals who were trained as recently as the first decade of the 2000s may have been taught to use a no-suicide contract that elicits promises from students that they will not kill themselves during a predetermined period of time. Although they are in widespread use and there is no evidence that they cause harm, there is *no evidence* that no-suicide contracts actually reduce suicide attempts, and these contracts *do not guarantee student safety*. In addition, there are concerns that these contracts can actually increase a school's liability with potentially suicidal clients. Safety plans, on the other hand, are put in place to help students know what to do when they have suicidal ideation or an increase in suicidal risk. They provide students with a concrete set of strategies to use when they start thinking about suicide.

Most safety plans include a step-by-step individualized process that the student and the mental health professional develop together. The more the safety plan is crafted in the student's words, with ideas and strategies that are based on the student's ideas, the more likely the plan is to be implemented. Professionals must take care not to impose ideas into the plan that the student is unlikely to carry out.

There are many examples of safety plans available online. Each plan, however, should be personalized to the individual student, with that student's internal coping strategies, external support people, and local resources. Each plan should include local and national suicide hotline numbers, including textlines, and a reminder to call 911 in an emergency. Finally, the safety plan should be signed and dated.

Practical strategy (schools): For years, the protocol for safety plans has been to give a hard copy to the students (as well as the parents and the school). In recent years, we have had students take a picture of their safety plan and save it to an easily accessed private folder on their phone. That is far easier than asking them to hold onto a piece of paper! In the past decade or so, we have also asked students to read aloud their safety plan into their phone. We have learned that hearing students say these steps, to themselves, in their own voice, when they are feeling calm and in control, can be very powerful. It might sound something like this: "Okay, XX, if you are listening to this, then that means that you are starting to feel anxious or upset. Remember, we have a plan for this, and the first step is XXX." As the student moves through the plan, they listen to "step 2" recorded on their phone, which may sound like this: "Okay, XX, now you are listening to step 2, which means that you are starting to feel even worse, and the things that you did in step 1 didn't work. Now it's time for us to reach out to our support system. Remember, we identified three people who can be supportive, so let's think about which one to talk to who can help." It will take some coaching and help, but hearing this plan in their own voice is powerful. Students will often try to get us to record it for them, but we know that this is not nearly as useful during the crisis itself. We know that it is hard to negate the power of our own voice.

Encourage the Use of Supportive Adjunctive Mental Health Resources . Not all students who return to school after a suicide or mental health crisis will continue to be under the care of an outside mental health professional, even if that is the recommended course of action. Students living in poverty, those who are marginalized or oppressed, those who live in rural communities, and those who live in unsupportive family environments are far less likely to have continued care.

Although school is not the place for ongoing intensive mental health treatment, telemental health care is one strategy to support students who have limited access to ongoing care. School-based telemental health care has been found to increase care and parent involvement in treatment for students living in areas with poor access to traditional mental health services. Other students benefit from resources such as mobile apps that support adolescent mental health and well-being, although there is currently very limited research about the effectiveness of this type of intervention for suicidal youth.

Students in Suicidal Crises

Intervening with students who are suicidal is incredibly complex. In general, this type of crisis counseling is *not* something that will be done in schools. Nevertheless, we conclude this chapter with a brief discussion of the type of crisis intervention counseling that is often done with individuals who are in a suicide crisis. We offer only a brief overview here and refer you to a full article about this type of intervention or other resources for more information. Nevertheless, we include this information because we believe that everyone working with students in suicide crisis should have a broad understanding of the steps that are generally included in crisis intervention counseling. When it comes to suicide prevention, preparedness and education are always worth the time and effort.

In general, the model for crisis intervention counseling with suicidal students is based on an expanded model of crisis intervention counseling (Figure 9.1; Granello, 2010). This model is intended to help already trained mental health professionals interact with students during times of high risk for suicide and *does not replace assessment by trained clinicians to determine appropriate levels of care and select appropriate intervention strategies.* These steps are intended only as a guide, and the needs of individual students may vary significantly. For example, specific cultural, developmental, or cognitive limitations of clients may shape the implementation of these strategies.

Step 1: Assess lethality
Step 2: Establish rapport
Step 3: Listen to the story
Step 4: Manage the feeling
Step 5: Explore alternatives
Step 6: Use behavioral strategies
Step 7: Follow up

Figure 9.1 Crisis Counseling With Potentially Suicidal Students
Source: Granello (2010).

Step 1: Assess Lethality

The first and most important step is to ensure the immediate safety of potentially suicidal students. This means never leaving the student alone, not even for a moment, not even to walk down the hall or make a quick phone call. Students should never be transported in a staff person's car or be allowed to leave the school building.

> *Practical strategy (schools): Schools should have in place a containment strategy. In other words, what steps will be taken if a highly suicidal student attempts to leave the school premises? Who will be informed? What is the number of the local police? Who will call the police? Who will notify parents? The time to answer these and other questions is now, not when a crisis is occurring. A completed containment strategy that is sitting on a shelf in someone's office isn't helpful either. Developing an active and readily available containment policy/procedure can help make students safer and mitigate risk.*

Step 2: Establish Rapport

The therapeutic relationship between the student and the helping professional is one of the best determinants for the outcome of a suicide crisis. Suicidal adolescents state that this relationship is one of the most, *if not the most*, helpful aspects of their treatment. Basic counseling skills and the Rogerian core conditions of warmth, empathy, congruence, and unconditional positive regard help convey a genuine, caring, and nonjudgmental therapeutic stance (Chiles & Strosahl, 2005).

Any interactions with suicidal students should be based in an approach that conveys calm and reassures the student that it is okay to talk about their suicidal thoughts and behaviors. We help students feel comfortable by saying things such as "It's okay. I know this is hard to talk about. Take your time. Use whatever words are most comfortable for you to describe what you are thinking and feeling." Even if we feel anxious about our own skills and overwhelmed by their story, a calm approach and matter-of-fact tone reassures students that we are able to help. In a time of crisis, having a strong, confident adult to lean on can be reassuring.

> *Practical strategy (self): Some simple, specific skills that help convey calm are to use short declarative sentences and downspeak. People in crisis cannot follow long or complex sentences. They need simple sentences that are easy to follow, even when they are distraught and distracted. Downspeak, where the pitch of the voice goes down at the end of sentences, results in declarative statements, whereas upspeak, the pattern that implies a question through a raised tone at the end of sentences, implies uncertainty and tentativeness. Upspeak can make students feel even more anxious and distressed. Listen to (or record) your own speech pattern or that of your peers to see if you can spot these differences. Downspeak, short sentences, and a slow pace communicate safety, control, and calm.*

Step 3: Listen to the Story

Students often tell us that every time they have tried to talk with an adult about their suicidal thoughts, they have been shut down. Well-meaning adults often minimize their stories. They are told, "That's ridiculous" or "Don't talk like that" or "S/he's not worth it." Other common responses to a declaration of suicidal intent include silence or changing the subject. As a result, although about 80% of young people who die by suicide or have an attempt tell someone they are suicidal in the weeks prior to their death, most have never had a chance to really fully tell their stories or fully process their emotions.

Practical strategy (schools): Of course, giving students time and space to tell their stories in school can be challenging. There is a press to move quickly and not spend too much time with any one student. There is a strategy that can help. We find when we say to students, "Tell me what is going on," we quickly get lost in the details of stories and people and endless iterations of "he said"/"she said" that don't help us get to the real point. Rather, we often say something like "It's okay. Take your time. Take a deep breath and think for a moment, and then <u>tell me what it is you want me to hear.</u>" That is a very different prompt—and we have found that it often yields <u>very</u> different (and much more meaningful) conversations.

Step 4: Manage the Feelings

Most people who are suicidal don't want to die. They simply want the pain to end. They feel a tremendous amount of psychological pain, and they can't imagine living with that pain another day. Because of the ambiguity that is frequently part of the crisis (i.e., not wanting to die but wanting the pain to end), it is not unusual for many different emotions to occur simultaneously, and suicidal individuals often feel overwhelmed by their emotions. Helping students to express their emotions is an important part of the healing process. Giving them space to cry, to express their anger, or to be scared teaches them that emotions are part of the human condition, and we don't have to cover them up. The goal is *not* emotional escalation. We don't want to "pour gasoline on the fire"—but we do want to encourage emotional expression. Statements such as "I know it feels overwhelming—this is a safe place for you to talk about these things" can be particularly helpful.

Practical strategy (schools): Consider teaching mindfulness skills. Mindfulness is gaining attention as an important psychological skill that allows people to stay immersed in stressful situations without becoming overwhelmed. Relaxation techniques and meditation can be important parts of mindfulness. Teaching students to focus on their experiences without judging them or equating these experiences to facts has been shown to help reduce cognitive distortions and feelings of anxiety (Chesin et al., 2018). Mindfulness skills can help give students a sense of control over their world and help them self-regulate their emotions. There are a multiple of smart phone apps that are available to help students learn, and use, these mindfulness skills.

Step 5: Explore Alternatives

Suicidal students have difficulty with problem-solving skills or finding options other than suicide to solve their problems. The developmental limitations of young people, who often have difficulty with problem-solving anyway, compound the dangers during times of suicide risk. Importantly, exploring alternatives is *not the same thing* as providing advice or answers, which is generally seen as minimizing or demeaning to those in crisis. Rather, developing a framework where the student works with the school staff member to develop a problem-solving strategy can be productive.

Practical strategy (schools): Motivational interviewing (MI) is a process that helps adolescents who are ambivalent about change (in this case, ambivalent about suicide) come to better understand their motivations for living. Without giving advice or telling the student what to do, MI uses empathy to help the student uncover underlying discrepancies between their goals and their behaviors and support the client's development of self-efficacy. MI has shown some initial promise as part of an overall approach to adolescent suicide intervention (Grupp-Phelan et al., 2019).

Step 6: Use Behavioral Strategies

Previously, we spoke about the importance of safety plans for helping students manage their suicidal crises. We believe that safety plans are extremely important and useful. We have also seen much success with something called a short-term positive action plan. In this strategy, students and mental health professionals develop a concrete, detailed plan that helps the student move forward in a specific area, rather than trying to make major changes or solve all the student's problems at once. Positive action plans recognize that small steps can have a great impact on the student's quality of life. People in crisis often feel overwhelmed by all of life's problems and can lose the ability to feel competent to make any positive headway about *anything*. As a result, all of their problems seem equally monumental. Helping students make small steps toward small goals helps them regain a sense of agency in their lives. Once they realize that they can start to make positive gains about very small goals, they start to see that they are able to take back some control. We have seen these positive action plans successfully used for *very small goals*. One student had an action plan to stack his books on the counter each night. Another had a plan to take a shower each Sunday. The point is, the successful completion of small goals matters.

Practical strategy (self): Just as with safety plans, short-term positive action plans can be recorded as voice messages into a student's phone. In fact, this is an option where it might make sense for anyone reading a book to give it a try to see how this works for yourself. Then, you can give a testimonial to your students if they tell you they think this sounds "stupid" or they don't think it will work. To start, think of a small goal and break it into its component parts. Read each of those parts into your phone, labeling each part in your phone as a step in the process. For example, one of us goes to the pool for a swim each morning, and sometimes we are busy, or it is cold, or we just don't want to go.

The positive action plan in my phone sounds like this: Step 1: "Okay, XX, if you are listening to this, then you don't want to go to the pool. So, step 1, find your water shoes. That's all. Just get your shoes." [Turn off phone.]. Step 2: "Ah, you're back. That means you still haven't found your motivation to go to the pool, but you have found your shoes. OK. Let me remind you what happens when you don't go to the pool. Let me remind you why this is important. As I remind you, why not take a moment, and put those shoes on your feet." You get the idea. Try it for yourself. After all, no one knows your excuses better than you, and no one knows how to argue with you better than you. So, the next time you have difficulty with one of your goals, give your "positive action plan" a try, and see how powerful it is to hear you giving yourself a pep talk! (And then see how easy it is to help students understand why this works.).

Step 7: Follow Up

Within the school setting, follow-up often involves ongoing meetings and interactions with the parents and the student. It may mean continuing contact with the outside referral agency. Regardless of the specific plan for an individual student, after each crisis situation, there is a great opportunity for school personnel to assess and evaluate the intervention strategies employed to make any necessary modifications or alterations for the future.

Practical strategy (schools): At least once per year, everyone involved in the Core Team for school-based suicide prevention, as well as everyone involved in the assessment and intervention of a suicidal student, should reflect on the experience. Look at the data. Collect all the information, notes, and feedback. Where is the learning? What can or should be done differently?

Conclusion

Working with suicidal students in schools involves specific and intentional planning by school mental health professionals. Because students who are in high-risk categories need a stable environment with clear expectations and supports, having clear plans and protocols in place prior to engaging with individual students is essential. Individual student plans always include parents and whenever possible and with appropriate releases signed, include appropriate outside mental health providers.

Students who require tier three, intensive interventions, typically are in one of three categories: students with on-going low-level suicide risk, students in suicide crisis, and students who return to school after they have been in out-patient treatment. In each of these instances, there are specific strategies that schools can use to support the mental health of their students.

References

American School Counselor Association. (2020). *The school counselor and suicide risk assessment*. https://www.schoolcounselor.org/

Centers for Disease Control and Prevention. (2012). *Parent engagement: Strategies for involving parents in school health*. U.S. Department of Health and Human Services.

Chesin, M. S., Brodsky, B. S., Beeler, B., Benjamin-Phillips, C. A., Taghavi, I., & Stanley, B. (2018). Perceptions of adjunctive mindfulness-based cognitive therapy to prevent suicidal behavior among high suicide-risk outpatient participants. *Crisis: The Journal of Crisis Intervention and Suicide Prevention, 39*(6), 451–460.

Chiles, J. A., & Strosahl, K. D. (2005). *Clinical manual for assessment and treatment of suicidal patients*. Washington, DC: American Psychiatric Press.

Diamond, G. M. (2014). Attachment-based family therapy interventions. *Psychotherapy, 51*, 15–19. doi:10.1037/a0032689

Giggie, M. A., Olvera, R. L., & Joshe, M. N. (2007). Screening for risk factors associated with violence in pediatric patients presenting to a psychiatric emergency department. *Journal of Psychiatric Practice, 13*(4), 246–252.

Granello, D. H. (2010). A suicide crisis intervention model with 25 practical strategies for implementation. *Journal of Mental Health Counseling, 32*(3), 218–35.

Grupp-Phelan, J., Stevens, J., Boyd, S., Cohen, D. M., Ammerman, R. T., Liddy-Hicks, S., Heck, K., Marcus, S. C., Stone, L., & Campo, J. V. (2019). Effect of a motivational interviewing–based intervention on initiation of mental health treatment and mental health after an emergency department visit among suicidal adolescents: A randomized clinical trial. *JAMA Network Open, 2*(12), e1917941. doi:10.1001/jamanetworkopen.2019.17941

Linehan, M. M. (1993). Dialectical behavior therapy for treatment of borderline personality disorder: implications for the treatment of substance abuse. *NIDA research monograph, 137*, 201–201.

Miller, A. L., Rathus, J. H., & Linehan, M. (2007). *Dialectical behavior therapy with suicidal adolescents.* Guilford Press.

Miller, W. R., & Rollnick, S. (2013). *Motivational interviewing: Helping people change* (3rd ed.). Guilford Press.

Singer, J. B., McManama, K. H., & LeCloux, M. (2017). Three psychotherapies for suicidal adolescents: Overview of conceptual frameworks and intervention techniques. *Child and Adolescent Social Work Journal, 34*, 95–106.

Substance Abuse Mental Health Services Administration. (2012). *Preventing suicide: A toolkit for high schools.* U.S. Department of Health and Human Services.

10

After a Suicide

Postvention in the School Environment

Sometimes, in spite of all of our best intentions and efforts, the students that we work so hard to care for and protect die by their own hand. It is a tragedy of unbelievable magnitude. And it is exactly what we have spent the last nine chapters of this book, and frankly, most of our professional careers, trying to avoid. When a student dies by suicide, in addition to managing our own grief and loss, we must do what mental health professionals so often must do during times of tragedy—try to help others even as we are suffering ourselves. We also know that we do this work with the very real understanding that other students in the building who have experienced this loss might now be at elevated risk for suicide themselves. A student death by suicide stretches everyone's ability to cope.

Schools play a pivotal role in the aftermath of a suicide by a student, staff member, or faculty member. In the days following a death, schools can become either a hotbed of rumor and speculation that can increase suicide risk or a place of safety where students can turn to trusted sources of information and support. In our own experiences as counselors and consultants to schools, we have seen both of these responses. We have seen schools grow into stronger and more caring environments after a suicide. Unfortunately, we have also witnessed the tragic results of inappropriate responses and copycat suicides. One of the key differences has been whether or not schools have in place, and follow, a suicide postvention strategy.

Suicide and Self-Injury in Schools. Darcy Haag Granello, Paul F. Granello, Gerald A. Juhnke,
Oxford University Press. © Oxford University Press 2023. DOI: 10.1093/oso/9780190059842.003.0010

The delivery of crisis response services in the aftermath of a youth suicide is referred to as suicide postvention. A comprehensive suicide postvention strategy that is developed *before the school is in the aftermath of a suicide* allows school staff to immediately implement guidelines that promote a healthy and safe environment. This means that during a crisis, there is no scrambling around to determine what to do. Rather, each member of the staff follows a predetermined protocol that is intentionally designed to limit risk.

Unfortunately, many of the best postvention strategies can be somewhat counterintuitive. That is, if left to our own devices and without the benefit of existing resources or research, many of us might implement strategies that could actually increase risk among students. Although, of course, none of us would ever raise risk intentionally, that could easily happen if we were left to make decisions on our own, particularly in the moment of crisis and chaos that occurs after a suicide. This is one of the major reasons advanced planning and preparation is essential.

Not long ago, we were called to assist in a postvention response at a school. (Please note that all identifying information, including information about the school, has been altered.) We received a call by a frantic vice principal at a religiously affiliated school after a second student died by suicide within a 2-month period. Previously, there had been no recorded incidents of student suicide in the school's more than 100-year history. Nevertheless, a Caucasian male junior died by suicide in early autumn, and a second Caucasian male junior took his own life less than 2 months later. Both boys used the same specific and unusual method, giving all indications of a copycat suicide. The school was uncertain of how to respond to the second suicide, and the school staff, faculty, and students were terrified that this would happen again. The administration felt guilty, wondering if they had inadvertently "caused" the second suicide. The students were angry, lashing out at their teachers for the "uncaring atmosphere" that was making students kill themselves. The sophomores were worried that there was something about their junior year that made students kill themselves. Rumors were rampant, text messaging was out of control, and by the time we arrived on campus the next day, there was an atmosphere of uncertainty and panic that was threatening to overtake the entire school.

As we listened to the administrators talk about their responses to the student deaths, it was clear that they did not have a postvention plan in place. After the death of the first student, the school went into grieving. As a religiously affiliated school, the administrators fell back on their faith to guide them. They held prayer vigils and candle lightings. They canceled classes for a school-wide memorial service in the school's chapel. They flew the flag at half-staff. Students also participated in developing mourning rituals. They made special pins for all the students to wear to remember the deceased student, and they put up a large banner of remembrance where all students could write their memories of the classmate they lost. On the surface, it would be easy to think that these responses were appropriate—even admirable. After all, they were sending a clear message to students that their school is a caring environment that mourns the death of one of its students and relies on faith to help them get through.

When the second student died by suicide weeks later, the administrators put a hold on all postvention activities and started searching the Internet to learn what they needed to do. They quickly learned that their responses to the first death may have inadvertently contributed to the death of the second student. But when they responded differently to the second death, the students became angry. They accused administrators of "being unfair." The first student who died was a popular athlete. The second student was less popular. The other students described him as a bit of a "loner." They said the school was "playing favorites" and they demanded another memorial service and prayer vigil. It was into this environment that we stepped onto campus to assist.

This case illustrates the critical role that postvention planning can play. As you will read in the following pages, many of the school's responses may indeed have contributed to the death of the second student. It is certainly unfair to "blame" the school—the student made an unfortunate and sad choice, and others are not responsible for that decision. It is certainly possible that he would have made the choice to die by suicide regardless of the school's response to the first suicide. However, there are things schools can do to *minimize* the risk of contagion, and it is certainly possible that a different response by the school could have led to a different outcome.

Four Major Goals in Any Postvention Response

Comprehensive suicide postvention plans outline specific actions that should be implemented in response to a suicide. These plans provide structure during difficult and potentially chaotic times. When schools develop a comprehensive suicide postvention strategy, there are four major goals that guide the process. Ultimately, a postvention strategy should (a) reduce the risk of suicide contagion, (b) provide the support needed to help survivors cope with a suicide death and express their grief, (c) address the social stigma associated with suicide, and (d) disseminate factual information (Brock, 2002). Throughout the process, school personnel must help students and staff members stay focused on learning and maintaining a healthy school environment.

Goal 1: Reduce the Risk of Suicide Contagion

Suicide contagion occurs when suicidal behavior is imitated. Also called "cluster suicides" or "copy-cat suicides," this type of suicide risk is relatively rare. However, when it does occur, it is most common in schools, among the elderly, and in close-knit communities, such as within police precincts or military units. It is difficult to say what motivates suicide contagion. However, among young people, guilt, overidentification with the deceased person, and modeling are all thought to play a role. Among teenagers, cluster or copycat suicides account for between 1% and 5% of all suicide deaths, resulting in 100–200 cluster suicides among teenagers each year (Zenere, 2009). There is evidence that the rate of cluster suicides among teenagers is increasing in the United States.

Practical strategy (schools): When someone their own age dies by suicide, it can threaten the adolescent sense of invulnerability. In other words, death suddenly becomes more "real" and suicide can start to seem like an "option." Some young people even talk about suicide feeling almost "inevitable"—like it is just something that "happens" to some people, and there is very little that can be done about it. It is clearly a dangerous and nihilistic belief that can keep these students from seeking help when they need it. Researchers are finding that more and more adolescents are responding to peer suicides with this sense of inevitability and doom. It is certainly something for school mental health professionals to watch for as they monitor student reactions to the suicide of one of their peers.

Clearly, for most students a single exposure to the suicidal behavior of another person, whether at the school or in the media, does not *in and of itself* result in imitative behavior. In other words, a student with no risk factors for suicide or pre-existing mental health problems is unlikely to become suicidal after the death of a classmate. Rather, it is the combination of that exposure and a predisposed psychological vulnerability that can result in increased risk for suicide contagion.

There are groups of students who may be at increased risk for suicide contagion. These include students who were in close contact with the deceased, such as team or club members, classmates who shared common schedules or activities, romantic interests, close friends, or others who perceive that they had something in common with the deceased student. Young people may overidentify with the deceased student if they believe they had similar life circumstances or experiences. In schools, this phenomenon has been observed following the suicide of a perceived leader, a popular student, or an athlete.

To reduce the potential of contagion, there are some specific strategies that schools should (or should not) employ.

Never Glamorize, Romanticize, or Glorify the Student or the Death. Locker memorials, flags at half-staff, planting a tree, and arm bands or specialized pins can inadvertently increase risk. In all schools, there are students who are psychologically vulnerable or who feel isolated or lonely, and who now see suicide as a way to gain "popularity" or "acceptance" within the school. Images that students have from the media or popular fiction can make suicide seem romantic or sensational, and witnessing these mourning rituals first-hand can play into those fantasies. Although students who wish to mourn the loss of a classmate by suicide may initially be angry or upset that they are not allowed to set up a locker memorial or wear special pins on their jerseys to honor that student, they typically understand the rationale for refraining from such activities when it is explained to them. Finally, just as it is important not to glamorize the student who died, however, neither should they be vilified. Instead, a message of "a good person who made a bad choice" is appropriate.

Practical strategy (schools): We know this is a difficult one. Students (and parents) often want to have a memorial of some type—and we often use the example of "planting a tree" for the student who died by suicide. If the school were to plant a tree for a student who died by suicide, what would they do if a student died in a car accident? Would they plant a tree? What if the student was drinking when they died? What if they were drinking and hit a car and killed another family? Suddenly, the school is making "moral" decisions about who is "tree-worthy"—and this is a bad place for schools to be. Making decisions ahead of time is always wise.

Do Not Announce the Student Death Over the Intercom or Other Public Address System. It is best if the death is announced in small groups, such as in a homeroom class, where teachers can follow predetermined protocols for announcing the death. In this way, teachers and staff can watch for extreme reactions from individual students, which may be indicative of increased risk.

Of course, unless the death has been confirmed as a suicide, the actual cause of death cannot be announced. Schools will need to have sample announcements prepared for (a) deaths confirmed as suicide and (b) deaths only deemed as suspicious but not confirmed as suicide. A standardized statement should be prepared that can be released to faculty so that it can be read to students, ensuring that all students receive the same information, ideally at the same time. These announcements must be clear and not overstate or assume facts that have not yet been provided. Finally, all announcements should be developmentally appropriate, with written information sent home to parents that includes additional information about common student reactions to suicide and/or sudden death of a classmate, how to respond, and information about suicide prevention.

Practical strategy (schools): Although announcing the student death in the morning should not be done over the loudspeaker, the American Foundation for Suicide Prevention (AFSP) has determined, and in our experience, we agree, that at the end of the first day, an announcement to the whole school is appropriate. A simple, short, and nonsensationalized message is best. For example, "Today has been a sad day for all of us. We encourage you to talk about ____'s death with your family, friends, or others in your life who can offer you support. We will have special staff here for you tomorrow to help you in dealing with our loss. For now, let us all take *a moment of silence for ___ " (AFSP & Suicide Prevention Resource Center [SPRC], 2018).*

Do Not Hold In-School Memorials or Cancel Classes or School. Again, the goal is to reduce the possibility that members of the school community overidentify with the deceased student or perceive that dying by suicide is a way to gain popularity within the school. In one high school nearby, the funeral service for a student who died by suicide was held in the school auditorium. The following year on the anniversary of the funeral, there was a copycat suicide. Within the last 2 years, there have been three more student suicides at the school.

We absolutely understand the desire of students—and often of parents—to hold these memorial services for students who die. We have been involved in many of these discussions. School administrators know they shouldn't hold these memorials, but there is no policy in place. Parents want to hold these memorials. We are brought in to try to negotiate the discussions. People are distraught, and emotions run high. We *cannot emphasize enough* the importance of having these protocols in place ahead of time. That way, these decisions are not made in the context of an individual—of someone's friend or a person's child. Instead, they are existing policies that are made for the safety of *all of the children in the school.*

Practical strategy (schools): We have found that holding an annual remembrance service for all students and all family members who died over the course of the year might be an option. This removes an individual student from any service—but gives the entire school a chance to hold a moment of remembrance and silence for students, faculty, staff and perhaps even parents and grandparents—indeed, everyone who was lost—without mentioning any names. This has to be done with care so that it is not "hijacked" into a memorial service for a particular student, but it may appease students and family to let them know that there will be a moment of silence for their loved one.

Never Discuss Suicide as a "Way to End Pain." We have said it before, but it is worth repeating: We NEVER say that a person killed themselves "because they were in so much pain" or "to make the pain go away." These are *extremely dangerous* statements to make. Suicide does not end pain. Suicide merely transfers the pain to those who are left behind. Suicide loss survivors are left with the burden and sadness of the suicide death for the rest of their lives. It is a natural thing for adults to try to explain a suicide death to a young person by saying something like "He was in such pain; he just couldn't go on. He killed himself as a way to end the pain." But that message can inadvertently teach young people that suicide is a way to make their pain go away.

Minimize Discussion of the Details of the Suicide Death. Students can ask a lot of questions, and it is easy to get caught up in the details of the death. Too many details can encourage contagion. Students learn from hearing the story of the student death, and copycat suicides can be the result of modeling the behaviors.

When a student focuses on the method of death, the best strategy is to answer the question simply and factually and then redirect the conversation to help them understand how the death has affected them and strategies that they can use to help cope with the loss (AFSP & SPRC, 2018). Students who focus on the details of the method may be having difficulties with processing their own loss and grief and be using the discussion about method to avoid talking about their feelings.

Practical strategy (schools): Be aware of the types of information— and misinformation—that students are sharing in the wake of a student suicide. Because much of this information is shared via social media, knowing what information is being shared and either posting accurate information (not about the specific suicide but about, for example, the link between mental illness and suicide), dispelling myths, or offering resources and information can be helpful. This is also when having peer educators (discussed in Chapter 7) can be useful, as peers can serve as helpful resources in the aftermath of a student suicide.

Clearly, the first and most important goal of the postvention protocol is to allow students to grieve in a way that minimizes the risk of suicide contagion. From this perspective, then, it is easy to see how many (well-intentioned) errors were made at the school with the two student suicides discussed at the beginning of the chapter. School officials had a school assembly and campus memorial service, canceling classes to encourage attendance. These events may have allowed the second student, who was unpopular and isolated, to begin to believe that the way to gain attention and acceptance at the school was through his own death. It is possible that the second student sat at those events and imagined what they might say about him or how his classmates might grieve his death. Additionally, the school allowed specific details of the student's death to be discussed at length, and the copycat suicide used the same, unique method of death. Next, students were allowed to set up memorials to the first student, with a specialized banner and pins. Again, for a segment of the student body, including perhaps the second student who died, this could have become an appealing way to "gain popularity or fame" within the school. While it is clear that none of these activities *caused* the death of the second student, it is possible that they inadvertently contributed to an atmosphere that made the possibility of suicide for that student more appealing.

When we met with student leaders at the school after the second death, many students were angry because they were not allowed to wear armbands or have special memorial pins for the second student. By this time, school officials had investigated appropriate postvention responses and learned that these types of memorials can unintentionally glamorize the student death. Students, however, thought the administration was being "unfair." They accused the school officials of "liking the first student better" or "trying to keep the students quiet" so parents of future students would not think poorly of the school. When we met with groups of students, we explained why these types of memorials, although well intentioned, could increase risk for their psychologically vulnerable classmates. Although most students understood and backed away from their original stance, one young woman got very angry. She challenged, "Are you telling me that because of the 5% of the students here who are psychologically unhealthy and might take it the wrong way, the 95% of us who are healthy can't have the memorials and services we want to have?" My answer? "Yes. That is *exactly* what I am saying." The reality is that those of us who are relatively psychologically healthy *do have a responsibility* to help protect and assist those of us who are not. It's a tough life lesson, but an important one. No one, not even this young woman, really *wants* to contribute to someone else's emotional pain. When she really stopped and thought about whether her right to wear a special pin or hang up a sign was really worth the possibility of losing another classmate to suicide, of course she reconsidered.

If a comprehensive suicide postvention plan had been in place before the first student suicide, of course, none of this would have happened. The administration would have had a consistent response to both student suicides, and students would have been given factual information and education about why the postvention choices were made.

Goal 2: Provide Support

Of course, the real reason the students were angry and upset after the second student suicide had very little to do with the administration or the school, and everything to do with the fact that they were feeling scared, guilty, angry, sad, and overwhelmed in general.

At least some of the students were looking for a person (or group) to lash out against in order to help make some sense of their mixed feelings. The idea that anger is displaced (e.g., expressed against another person or object rather than the true object of our feelings) is commonplace. We need only look at the child who is angry at a parent and kicks the dog or a person who is angry at his boss and punches his hand through a wall to see evidence of how this affects our lives. In this instance, the students had a lot of feelings, including anger toward the students who died by suicide. It is difficult to be angry at someone and sad because they are gone at the same time, and it may have been easier (or safer) to be angry at the administration (or some random expert) instead. Of course, school officials made some choices that caused the students to be angry, but at least some of the wrath they were experiencing had very little to do with these choices and very much to do with the chaotic and uncomfortable emotions the students were experiencing. A postvention response that helped students process their complicated emotions in appropriate ways would have helped students navigate this difficult grieving process.

Suicide bereavement differs from other types of grief. Most suicide loss survivors report feeling guilty and angry (at the person who died, at themselves, at others whom they perceive didn't offer help, at God, or at the world in general). In fact, compared to individuals who lost loved ones to homicide, accidents, or illness, suicide loss survivors experience the following:

- More intense grief reactions than any of the other survivor groups
- Greater likelihood of assuming responsibility for the person's death, believing they should have done something to prevent it
- More self-destructive behaviors
- Higher levels of shame and perceived rejection (Bailley et al., 1999; Silverman et al., 1994–95)

Practical strategy (reader): Although at the moment we are discussing how to navigate a <u>school</u> through a postvention process, the reality is that if you are reading this and going through the postvention process, you are navigating through this process too. We hope you take a moment to allow yourself time to grieve, cry, mourn, and experience all of the complex emotions that others are feeling too. We encourage you to seek professional help if you need it, and to understand that even those of us who help others need help too. We stand with you in this moment, and we share our heartfelt sympathy for your loss. Sadly, we know all too well what it feels like to walk with others through this journey as we walk the path ourselves.

After the loss of a student to suicide, classmates who knew that the student was at risk, knew about the suicide plans but kept them a secret, or became the "self-appointed therapist" to the suicidal student are at increased risk for suicide themselves. This is particularly problematic because research demonstrates that the majority of young people who know a peer is suicidal do not take appropriate steps to intervene. In fact, although more than 80%% of teenagers who die by suicide tell someone they plan to kill themselves and 90% demonstrate clear warning signs, only 25% of teenagers say they would tell an adult if they knew a peer was suicidal (Helms, 2003). As a result, after a suicide, there may be many members of the student body who are grieving intensely and who are at increased risk for suicide themselves. These individuals need extra support and assistance to work through the grieving process. In general, postvention strategies must include several different mechanisms for emotional support. Students who need immediate assistance must be given easy access to counseling and care, and ongoing help must be available (either at the school or through identified off-campus providers).

Practical strategy (schools): In the aftermath of a student suicide, a structured protocol typically includes multiple strategies to help students cope. These strategies recognize that students will have different reactions to the loss and will need a variety of strategies over the ensuing days, and possibly weeks, to help them navigate the complex emotions they may be experiencing. It is important to reach out to students in intentional and specific ways, such as during homerooms or with interventions designed specifically for the groups of students most directly affected by the loss. All students should be provided the opportunity for small group meetings and individual counseling to process their reactions to the death and to obtain support (for more information and strategies, see AFSP & SPRC, 2018).

Goal 3: Address Social Stigma

As we have said repeatedly throughout this book, suicide is surrounded by stigma and taboo. In the aftermath of a suicide, that stigma can get mixed up with the specifics of the death of an individual student, making a bad situation worse. Stories, rumors, gossip, and hearsay collide with the existing stigma, and before long, very bad things are being said about the student who has died. It is difficult to stop. We know it. Working to address the stigma of mental health and suicide before, and after, a death is critical. We take care not to have any of the messaging tied to any student or any death. We just reinforce the same consistent messages that we have been giving to the students all along: Mental illness is an illness like any other. Get help. Get help for a friend. Reach out. Ask, RU OK? Nothing changes after a student death. The messages remain the same.

Practical strategy (schools): Sometimes, in the aftermath of a student suicide, stories circulate about the events that led up to the suicide, and the result is that very simplistic answers are used to

*explain the death. (You might recall the stories in Chapter 3 of the
student who wanted a pizza or the young man who was sent home
from baseball practice as examples of seemingly simplistic "reasons"
these young people died by suicide.) Similarly, other students might
start to assume that what they have heard about suicide—that
many students who die by suicide have pre-existing underlying
conditions (a mental illness, social isolation, or bullying)—automatically applies to the student who died. They may begin to craft
stories or narratives about the deceased student with very little information or evidence. In all cases, suicide prevention messaging
should stay consistent to what was in place prior to the death.
Whatever campaigns existed in the school prior to the death should
remain in place. Otherwise, students can (and often will) make
assumptions that any changes to these campaigns are in response to
the circumstances of the recent death.*

Goal 4: Provide Information

After a suicide, it is tempting to rush in with suicide prevention
programming. We often get calls from schools right after a student
death, asking us to develop a suicide prevention program for the
school. We understand the temptation, but it is poorly timed. In the
aftermath of a student death, we gently say, "Now is not the time."
There will be plenty of time to set up a comprehensive suicide prevention program in the weeks and months that follow.

But all of this doesn't mean that suicide shouldn't be discussed at
all. We are not suggesting that a student's death should be kept quiet
or students should be kept in the dark—quite the contrary. Schools
should provide students with facts about suicide risk and mental
health resources. This should be done in small groups, or individually, if needed. The adults in the school shouldn't be afraid to talk
about suicide and to directly ask students if they are okay, or if they
are thinking about suicide. The point is only that in the aftermath

of a student suicide, starting a suicide prevention program can feel insensitive and callous to the other students. It can put the focus of the suicide prevention campaign on the student who died, which can inadvertently derail the efforts of the entire campaign.

After a student death, we recommend that the school mental health professionals focus on taking care of the students, staff, and teachers. Provide emotional support, limit contagion, address the social stigma that prevents people from getting the help they need, and give people some basic information about how to get help.

Practical strategy (schools): In the aftermath of a suicide, the most important thing is to provide basic information on the following:
- *Healthy coping strategies, such as exercise, relaxation, or spending time with friends or family*
- *Ways to manage loss and grief, such as identifying and expressing emotions, focusing on the future, or thinking of ways to remember the person who died (within the guidelines of the school's policy for memorials)*
- *Strategies to get through a crisis, such as talking to a counselor or calling a crisis line*
- *What do if you or someone you know is feeling suicidal, including listing all of the school-based and local supports and hotline information*

The Postvention Protocol

A suicide postvention protocol involves a *set of written procedures and guidelines* that are developed before a suicide occurs. These should be disseminated widely so everyone knows and understands their roles and responsibilities and can act on a moment's notice. A postvention team that has been well trained and is prepared to step up and implement the protocol is essential. The AFSP has teamed up with the SPRC to develop a toolkit for schools for postvention (AFSP & SPRC, 2018). We highly recommend that schools make use of this valuable and free resource.

The following steps are general guidelines only and are adapted from a variety of sources, including the AFSP and SPRC (2018) guidelines, the School-Based Youth Suicide Prevention Guide (Doan et al., 2003), the Maine Youth Suicide Prevention Program (DiCara et al., 2009), and the work of Brock (2002), as well as our own experiences working with schools in the aftermath of a student suicide.

1. Before a crisis occurs, establish a crisis response team. Many school districts already have such a team in place, and it is important to know if such a team exists, and if so, how to interact appropriately with the existing resources. Crisis response teams typically involve both school and community resources.

   - Crisis teams are typically kept rather small—fewer than 10 people—so they can mobilize quickly. They often involve the school mental health professionals, school administrators, and perhaps a person who has expertise in technology who can help with disseminating important messages quickly. It may also be helpful to have a member of the community crisis response network on the team, if the school will be bringing in members of the community to help students navigate the immediate mental health crisis.

2. Contact the police, coroner's office, or local hospital to the verify the death and get the facts.

   - It is essential that the suicide be officially confirmed before there is any public disclosure or speculation of suicide by any personnel in the school. It is often difficult to conclude a cause of death, and a determination of suicide must be made by a medical examiner or coroner. Even the most obvious cases of suicide should never be classified as such without official designation. Even if the death has officially been classified as a suicide, however, we strongly urge schools to never release the cause of death as a suicide unless the family members agree. Consider this story:

One of us had a difficult conversation recently with a young person who was angry that in the days after a student death the school continued to call the death an "accident," when all of the students agreed (and medical reports appeared to confirm) that it was a suicide. The student was a suicide prevention peer educator in the school, yet she was outspoken in her anger, stating that the school was trying to "look good" by denying the suicide. The students in school were becoming angry and frustrated that the school was refusing to call the death a suicide. I took her aside, and explained that we needed her help. I told her that the parents simply were not ready to classify the death as a suicide. I tried to help her understand what it must be like to lose a child, how difficult it would be to grieve that death, and how terrible it must be to have others tell you that it was a suicide. I told her that the school simply couldn't force the parents to label this death a suicide when they weren't ready. She started to understand. Then I said that neither I nor the school officials could possibly stand up and explain to the students *why* we weren't classifying the death as suicide. We couldn't explain this to the students—but *she could*. I asked her for her help. She immediately agreed. She, and her fellow peer educators, started changing the narrative in the school. It was powerful. She became engaged in raising the empathy of the entire student body, and she became an important advocate for the program. Ultimately, the family was ready to declare the student death a suicide, *in their own time*, and the students learned a valuable lesson. It was an important lesson for the school too about how having student leaders in suicide prevention in place *before a moment of crisis* became a critical tool that could be deployed during times of crisis.

3. Inform the school superintendent and administrators of schools where siblings are enrolled.
4. Contact the family of the deceased student to express condolences.
5. Notify and activate the school's crisis response team.
   - Use a predetermined approach (texting, phone calls) that allows for *direct communication* with the crisis response team.
   - Be sure each member of the crisis response team follows individual specific crisis response duties (e.g., crisis response coordinator, media liaison, medical liaison, security liaison, liaison with the family) that have been preassigned to each team member.
   - Operationalize the plan for communicating the news to students and parents.
6. Ensure that the entire protocol addresses cultural diversity.
   - All postvention responses must be appropriate for the culture of the deceased, as well as for those who are grieving. People from different cultures respond differently to suicide, death, and grieving.
   - When necessary, engage "cultural brokers" to act as liaisons between the family, community, and school when key members of the school staff are not from the same culture as the student who died by suicide or as students who are struggling to cope with the loss.
7. Schedule a time and place to notify faculty members and staff.
   - If possible, set up a meeting before the start of the school day.
   - Prepare school personnel for possible student reactions.

- Remember support staff (e.g., kitchen staff, custodians, bus drivers, secretaries) and any substitute teachers.
- Allow time for staff to ask questions and express feelings.
- Clarify the prearranged steps that will be taken to support school personnel, students, and parents (e.g., grief counseling, debriefing).
- Remind staff of the possibility of suicide contagion. Reinforce the necessity of following the postvention guidelines in order to minimize the potential for contagion.
- Ask the staff to identify any concerns they may have about individual students. Clarify how to monitor at-risk students.

8. Activate procedures for responding to media.
   - Announce how the school will interact with media representatives.
   - Remind staff not to talk with the press, spread rumors, or repeat stories. All inquiries must be directed to the designated media spokesperson.
   - Reinforce that specific media guidelines are in place to help minimize contagion.
   - Remember to monitor social media accounts, as necessary, to watch for the possibility of contagion.

9. Contact community support services, local mental health agencies, other school counselors, and clergy to arrange for crisis intervention assistance, if previously arranged.
   - Be prepared to identify and refer students who are most likely to be at high risk because of their close physical and emotional contact with the deceased student. Consider siblings, students who may identify with the deceased student, team members, friends, romantic interests, and anyone who was considered to be at risk for suicide prior to the death (e.g., those with pre-existing mental illness who lack coping skills or support systems).

10. Announce the death to students through a prearranged system.

   - Make the announcement in person, in small groups or classroom settings. If possible, all students should be given the same information at the same time (such as in a homeroom situation) by teachers or other adults they know and trust.

   - Teachers and others making the announcement should be provided with a written list of procedures for announcing the suicide to students and for identifying students who may need additional support.

   - The announcement should be honest and direct, including only the facts as they have been officially communicated. If the death has not yet been officially classified as a suicide, simply acknowledge that the cause is unknown.

   - Allow time for initial reactions and discussion, but limit details of the death.

   - Frame suicide as a poor choice, not as a way to end pain.

   - Use words such as "suicide death" or "completed suicide" rather than "committed suicide" or "successful suicide."

11. For safety purposes, be very careful about allowing students to leave school unattended.

   - Students should be encouraged to stay in school and maintain a regular school routine.

   - Implement an enhanced system to carefully track student attendance, and allow students to leave school premises only with parental permission.

   - If the safety of a student who has left the building without permission is a significant concern and the parents cannot be reached, contact the police.

12. Provide written information for parents/guardians as soon as possible so they can be prepared and available to provide support to their children.

- The notification should include information about how the school is responding to the crisis as well as resources and information on youth suicide prevention, local referrals, and specific person(s) at the school to contact with questions or for more information.
- Consider parent meeting(s) or other strategies to disseminate more information or to allow parents to ask questions about how to help their grieving children.
- Provide parents (and other caregivers) with developmentally appropriate tips for talking about suicide, death, and grieving, as well as specific resources if their child needs further counseling or if they believe their child might be suicidal.

13. Have crisis team available in the deceased student's classes.
    - Follow the deceased student's schedule to observe reactions of students and to follow up, if necessary.

14. Establish support stations and counseling rooms and publicize their availability for students.
    - Be sure to document who attends and the time of their attendance. Follow up with these students, as needed.

15. Make sure administrators and staff are visible in hallways and during lunch to monitor students and provide a calming presence for the school.

16. Provide secretaries or others who answer the phone with a prepared script to field telephone calls or to answer inquiries from people who show up at the school.

17. Use a prearranged strategy to monitor and assist students who may be at increased risk for suicide.
    - Provide additional suicide loss survivor support services and education about suicide bereavement.
    - Follow up with these students (and their families, as necessary) for as long as needed.
    - Make sure all students have access to suicide hotline numbers.

- Provide extra support through special events (e.g., anniversaries, special events, transitions), which can be particularly difficult for students to manage after a suicide death.
- Give on-going special attention to students in peer groups, friends, teams, romantic partners, and others who may be at higher risk. They should be encouraged to talk about their reactions. Attention to these students during the postvention period may help limit future suicidal behavior.

18. Conduct daily debriefing with faculty and staff during the initial crisis and postvention periods.
19. Reschedule any immediate stressful academic exercises or tests, but try to stay with the general school schedule as much as possible.
    - Keep the school open, and follow regular school routines to the extent possible.
    - Although the school must be attentive to those who are grieving, it is important to remember that not all students were equally affected by the death.
    - Convey the message that while we all grieve, life must go on.
20. Provide information about the funeral to students and parents.
    - Work with family and ask, if possible, if the funeral service can be held after school hours. If this is not possible, allow students to attend the funeral with parental permission and announce the policy regarding school absence for funeral attendance.
    - Avoid use of the school as a site for the funeral. Not only can this glorify the student death, but also it can increase the likelihood that some young people will forever identify the room in which the service is held with death.
21. Offer ongoing grief counseling for students and staff.

- Provide opportunities to process the grief, recognizing that for some students, this is the first time they have encountered death.
- Allow students to express their feelings, but take care not to give the death so much attention that it may make the idea of suicide attractive to other vulnerable students. This delicate balance will require a thoughtful and considered approach.

22. Follow up with students identified as at risk. Maintain follow-up as long as possible.
    - Use outside referral sources for students who need more care than the school can (or should) provide.
23. Carefully monitor memorial activities or events.
    - Appropriate commemorative activities must be carefully selected to minimize the possibility of glamorizing the suicide.
    - Instead of memorial activities, encourage donations to a charity or to community-based (as opposed to school-based) youth suicide prevention efforts, such as fielding a team for a suicide prevention walk. Although students and grieving families may insist that their deceased loved ones be honored, channeling the energy into constructive events that help the living is most productive.
    - Advance planning regarding memorializing student deaths is strongly recommended. This guards against giving students who die by suicide more (or less) attention than students who die by other means. This includes dedication pages in student yearbooks and newspapers, where space provided and information contained within the dedication should be consistent. Many school yearbook publishers offer well-thought-out guidelines for dedication pages. Overall, with all student memorials, a fair and equitable policy eliminates the possibility that popular students or those who die by certain types of death

will garner more attention, and a policy developed in advance can help school personnel stay with school procedure, rather than being driven by the intensity of emotions during a time of crisis.

24. Follow the prearranged protocol for emptying the student's locker and returning personal items to the family. Allow the family to determine whether they wish to do this in private or have the school return the items to them. If family wishes to empty the locker, provide a quiet time and support to meet their wishes.

25. Determine how diplomas, athletic letters, or other awards will be given posthumously. Plan ahead and develop a school policy for how graduation and award ceremonies will be handled. If, for example, the school will award honorary diplomas, the criteria should be determined in advance to provide consistency and fairness to all students.

26. Get support for the crisis response team, allowing them to debrief from the secondary trauma of the postvention period.

27. Document activities as dictated by school protocols.
    • Use learning and experiences to update the suicide postvention protocol for the future.

The Special Case of a Teacher or Staff Member Suicide

Although we have been focusing on the loss of a student to suicide, there are also times when schools lose a staff member or teacher to suicide. Although the overall protocols look similar, we also know that there are some differences in how students—and teachers and staff members—react to the loss. There is, sadly, very little research on how to help schools navigate this extremely difficult loss. We only know from our experience that helping students, staff, and other teachers navigate the suicide of a teacher or staff member takes extra time and gentle guidance. Although the steps in the process are the same, we recognize that schools should be prepared for the grieving process to be longer and more complicated, especially since the people who are guiding the process are likely to be deeply embedded in their own grieving process. In the special case of the death of a teacher or staff member to suicide, we *highly recommend* that from the very start schools bring in an outside specialist who is an expert in suicide grieving to help everyone navigate the process.

Working With the Media

Unfortunately, suicide can be a newsworthy event. This is even more true when the person who died was young. After a suicide, it is extremely likely that the suicide death will be reported, particularly in rural areas or small towns. However, research has demonstrated that how the media covers a suicide death has a significant influence on suicide contagion. The recognition of the role of the media began in the 1980s, after a suicide death by a man who jumped in front of a subway train in Vienna, Austria. Following the death, television reporters engaged in a series of dramatic and sensational stories of the suicide that culminated in a re-enactment of the suicide on the evening news. Over the following weeks and months, there were a series of copycat suicides on the same subway tracks. It became clear that the news reporting itself was increasing the risk for suicide. An alternative media campaign was put into place, and within 6 months, subway suicides and nonfatal attempts dropped by more than 80%. Importantly, *all suicide deaths*, not just subway deaths, decreased significantly (Etzersdorfer & Sonneck, 1998).

In the subsequent decades, we have learned much about the ways the media can minimize (or encourage) the possibility of suicide contagion (AFSP, American Association of Suicidology [AAS], &

Annenberg Public Policy Center [APPC], n.d.). In fact, implementation of recommendations for media coverage of suicide has been
shown to decrease suicide rates. Further, research finds an increase
in suicide by readers or viewers when

- the number of stories about individual suicides increases,
- a particular death is reported at length or in many stories,
- the story of an individual death by suicide is placed on the
  front page or at the beginning of a broadcast, or
- the headlines about specific suicide deaths are dramatic (such
  as a relatively recent example: "Boy, 10, Kills Himself Over
  Poor Grades").

The power of the media clearly can impact suicide and suicide
prevention. Responsible handling of suicide by the media can
help inform readers and viewers about the likely causes of suicide,
its warning signs, trends in suicide rates, and recent treatment
advances. Although media stories about individual deaths by suicide may be newsworthy and need to be covered, they also have the
potential to do harm if proper protocol is not followed.

When the suicide of a young person occurs, schools are often
the first place the media will go for information. Thus, it is essential that working with the media and proper media guidelines for
reporting a student death by suicide be included in the postvention
protocols.

It is important to note that just like the young woman discussed
earlier who needed to have the rationale for the decision not to
hold a memorial service following the second student suicide
explained to her, it is clear that most journalists want to do the right
thing and have no desire to encourage suicide contagion through
their reporting. In fact, most people want to do the right thing, and
it is the responsibility of everyone involved in suicide prevention
to share education and prevention protocols with others, including
the media.

A story from the life of one of the authors illustrates the point:

Our house is in a suburban setting on the outskirts of a large mid-western city. Our backyard faces a small city park, and on the other side of the park sits both a middle and a high school. One afternoon, a man rode his bike into the park just before school was released, walked into the small woods, and shot himself. Students leaving the school building heard the gunshot, and several young people walking through the park on the way home from school found the body and called 911 on their cell phones. Within minutes, the park was filled with police cars, fire trucks, and emergency personnel. Students were rounded up and put in the park shelter to wait to be interviewed by police. They were frightened and shocked by their experience. Before long, the streets of our otherwise quiet neighborhood were filled with satellite television trucks, newspaper reporters, and other members of the media. Everyone was excited to get the "scoop" about the young, privileged suburban students, innocently walking home from school, who had such a terrifying encounter with death. Parents rushed into the park to be with the children, and before long, it was chaos. I could witness all of this from the deck in our backyard, and I was angered by what I saw. The students were being interviewed one by one by the police, and once released from these official interviews, they were surrounded by television cameras and microphones. Rather than sit fuming, I went upstairs to my home office and printed out several copies of the media guidelines for reporting on suicide, took them to the park, and began distributing copies. I spoke with anyone who would listen about the harmful effects of sensationalizing this story. I spoke about the potential for suicide contagion and the potential to make the students who found the body into unwilling "celebrities" in their school. I reminded every reporter I spoke with that the possibility of an exciting story was certainly not worth the potential of another death. The reporters listened. They understood. Most of the reporters took copies of the guidelines to bring back to their newspapers and television studios. That evening, I surfed through all the evening news programs on the local television channels and heard nothing about the suicide. The next day, buried on a back page of the metro section of the newspaper, was a small story of an unidentified man who shot himself in a local park. There was no mention of the nearby schools nor the students who found the body.

I learned a very, very valuable lesson that day. If we want responsible media reporting of suicide, then it is our responsibility to educate the members of the media. And most of the time, they listen. All of us must recognize that suicide prevention is a shared responsibility, and we must all do our part.

The following guidelines can assist schools in their work with the media following a student suicide. These guidelines are based upon those formulated by the AFSP, AAS, and SPRC (n.d.) and Granello and Granello (2007):

In general, the school official appointed by the school to work with the media *should* do the following:

- Have an established set of procedures in place *prior to the suicide* to interact with the media during the postvention time period.
- Write down key points before talking with reporters and have some basic information about the school ready to share with reporters.
- Express appropriate concerns for the deceased student's family members.
- Provide appropriate factual information (typically age and grade).
- Acknowledge the suicide (if it has been officially ruled a suicide by a medical examiner), but avoid discussion of details of the death (method, location).

- Encourage reporters to provide information that increases public awareness of risk factors and warning signs rather than focuses on the suicide.
- Provide information about local and school-based resources for suicide prevention and crisis intervention.
- Share with reporters information about media guidelines for reporting on suicide and discuss the dangers of suicide contagion.
- Encourage placement of the story within the inside pages of the newspaper (or lower in media feeds) or later in the television news broadcast, rather than the headlines or lead story.
- Frame suicide and the deceased person as a "good person who made a bad choice." Acknowledge that suicide is complex and there are no simplistic reasons people make this choice. Include positive aspects of the student's life to provide a more balanced picture and decrease overidentification with the student by peers.

In general, the school official appointed by the school to work with the media *should not* do the following:

- Present an overly simplistic explanation for the suicide. Suicide is never the result of a single factor or event.
- Sensationalize, romanticize, or glorify the suicide.
- Use a picture of the student who died by suicide.
- Use the word "suicide" in the headline of the article.
- Dramatize the impact of the suicide through descriptions or pictures of grieving friends, families, teachers, or classmates. This could encourage contagion.
- Allow peers or classmates on TV or in print media to tell stories of their own experiences with suicide or suicide attempts. This could lead to overidentification.
- Provide details or descriptions of the suicide.
- Describe suicide as a "way to end the pain."

A complete copy of the protocol "Reporting on Suicide, Recommendations for the Media" is available through the AFSP.

Finally, school newspapers can provide a positive venue for sharing information about appropriate help seeking and resources. Many school newspapers (and parent newsletters) provide information about student mental health as well as suicide risk factors and warning signs. In the weeks and months after a completed suicide, it is important to keep this information available for students. Newspaper articles need not refer directly to the suicide but can simply be "healthy reminders" of how to maintain optimal mental health and where to go to find assistance. For example, before exams, or before the start of a break from school (e.g., winter holidays or summer vacation), student and parent newsletters can provide a story of "managing stress" to include important resources. At our universities, whenever there is a student suicide, the student newspaper makes no mention of the death but runs an "informational article" on help seeking and mental health resources. In this way, students who are not aware of the death are not given information about it, but those who are aware (or who are feeling emotionally vulnerable for *any* reason) are reminded that there are those on campus who are willing and available to help. These types of articles and "public service announcements" should be an ongoing part of every school's media campaign.

Concluding Note

Suicide postvention is a critical component of school-based suicide prevention, yet it is often misguided and handled poorly. All too often, school personnel wait until a student dies by suicide and then scramble to try to make good choices. In this context, it is almost inevitable that mistakes will occur, and the consequences of those mistakes can be devastating. If you are working in a school right now, investigate the school's policies and procedures regarding suicide postvention, and if none are in place (or if they are out-dated), update them now. It is one of the most important things you can do to help your school be a place that limits the potential for suicide contagion.

References

American Foundation for Suicide Prevention, American Association of Suicidology, & Annenberg Public Policy Center. (n.d.). *Reporting on Suicide, recommendations for the media.* http://www.afsp.org

American Foundation for Suicide Prevention & Suicide Prevention Resource Center. (2018). *After a suicide: A toolkit for schools* (2nd ed.). Education Development.

Bailley, S. E., Kral, M. J., & Dunham, K. (1999). Survivors of suicide do grieve differently: Empirical support for a common sense proposition. *Suicide and Life Threatening Behavior, 29,* 256–271.

Brock, S. E. (2002). School suicide postvention. In S. E. Brock, P. J. Lazarus, & S. R. Jimerson (Eds.), *Best practices in school crisis prevention and intervention* (pp. 211–224). National Association of School Psychologists.

DiCara, C., O'Halloran, S., Williams, L., & Brooks, C. C. (2009). *Maine Youth Suicide Prevention Program.* https://www.maine.gov/suicide/docs/Guidelines%2010-2009--w%20discl.pdf

Doan, J., Roggenbaum, S., & Lazear, K. (2003). *Youth suicide prevention school-based guide—Issue brief 7a: Preparing for and responding to a death by suicide: Steps for responding to a suicidal crisis* (FMHI Series Publication #218-7a). Department of Child and Family Studies, Division of State and Local Support, Louis de la Parte Florida Mental Health Institute, University of South Florida.

Etzersdorfer, E., & Sonneck, G. (1998). Preventing suicide by influencing mass-media reporting. The Viennese experience 1980–1996. *Archives of Suicide Research, 4,* 67–74.

Granello, D. H., & Granello, P. F. (2007). *Suicide: An essential guide for helping professionals and educators.* Allyn & Bacon.

Helms, J. F. (2003). Barriers to help-seeking among 12th graders. *Journal of Educational and Psychological Consultation, 14*(1), 27–40.

Silverman, E., Range, L., & Overholser, J. (1994–1995). Bereavement from suicide as a compared to other forms of bereavement. *Omega, 30,* 41–51.

Zenere, F. J. (2009, October 1). Suicide clusters and contagion. *Principal Leadership Magazine.*

Index

For the benefit of digital users, indexed terms that span two pages (e.g., 52–53) may, on occasion, appear on only one of those pages.